Relief from Hot Flashes

Also by Gary Elkins PhD, ABPP, ABPH

*Hypnotic Relaxation Therapy: Principles
and Applications*

Relief from Hot Flashes

The Natural, Drug-Free Program to Reduce Hot Flashes, Improve Sleep, and Ease Stress

Gary Elkins, PhD, ABPP, ABPH

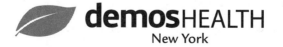

demosHEALTH
New York

Visit our website at www.demoshealth.com

ISBN: 978-1-936303-56-4
e-book ISBN: 978-1-617051-91-3

Acquisitions Editor: Julia Pastore
Compositor: diacriTech

Medical information provided by Demos Health, in the absence of a visit with a health care professional, must be considered as an educational service only. This book is not designed to replace a physician's independent judgment about the appropriateness or risks of a procedure or therapy for a given patient. Our purpose is to provide you with information that will help you make your own health care decisions.

The information and opinions provided here are believed to be accurate and sound, based on the best judgment available to the authors, editors, and publisher, but readers who fail to consult appropriate health authorities assume the risk of injuries. The publisher is not responsible for errors or omissions. The editors and publisher welcome any reader to report to the publisher any discrepancies or inaccuracies noticed.

Library of Congress Cataloging-in-Publication Data

Elkins, Gary Ray, 1952-
  Relief from hot flashes : the natural, drug-free program to reduce hot flashes, improve sleep, and ease stress / Gary Elkins, Ph.D., ABPP, ABPH.
      pages cm
  Includes bibliographical references and index.
  ISBN 978-1-936303-56-4
  1. Menopause—Treatment—Popular works. 2. Middle-aged women—Health and hygiene—Popular works. I. Title.
  RG186.E555 2014
  618.1′75—dc23
                                                          2014000387

Special discounts on bulk quantities of Demos Health books are available to corporations, professional associations, pharmaceutical companies, health care organizations, and other qualifying groups. For details, please contact:

Special Sales Department
Demos Medical Publishing, LLC
11 West 42nd Street, 15th Floor
New York, NY 10036
Phone: 800-532-8663 or 212-683-0072
Fax: 212-941-7842
E-mail: specialsales@demosmedpub.com

Printed in the United States of America by McNaughton & Gunn.
14 15 16 17 18 / 5 4 3 2 1

For Guillerma,
Forever and Always

Contents

Foreword by Patricia J. Sulak, MD   *ix*
Preface   *xi*
Acknowledgments   *xv*

UNDERSTANDING HOT FLASHES

1. How This Book Will Help You   *3*
2. What Causes Hot Flashes?   *15*
3. Breast Cancer and Hot Flashes   *23*
4. Hormone Replacement: The Risks and Benefits   *33*
5. Nonhormonal Therapies for Hot Flashes:
   What Do We Really Know?   *45*
6. Hypnotic Relaxation Therapy: What It Is and
   Why You Need It   *63*

FIRST THINGS FIRST

7. Measuring Your Hot Flashes   *75*
8. Identifying Your Hot Flash Triggers   *87*
9. Assessing Your Sleep   *95*
10. Rating the Interference of Your Hot Flashes on
    Your Mood, Relationships, and Quality of Life   *101*

HYPNOTIC RELAXATION THERAPY: THE SOLUTION FOR HOT FLASHES

11. Hypnotic Relaxation Therapy: What Happens   *111*
12. Week 1: Starting Your Practice   *119*
13. Week 2: Individualizing Your Practice   *129*
14. Week 3: Learning Self-Hypnosis for Hot Flashes   *147*
15. Week 4: Knowing Your Body and Controlling
    Your Hot Flashes   *163*
16. Week 5: Setting Goals and Maintaining
    Your Progress   *179*

CONTENTS

17. Assessing Your Progress   **195**
18. If You Need Additional Help   **209**

Afterword: Women Share Their Experiences Using
    the Relief from Hot Flashes *Program*   217
Appendix
    Hot Flash Daily Diary   225
    Hot Flash Triggers log   227
    Sleep Rating Form   229
    Hot Flash Related Daily Interference Scale (HFRDIS)   231
    Hypnotic Relaxation Practice Checklist   233
Bibliography   235
Index   251

Foreword

Hot flashes and night sweats are a common occurrence in menopausal women and breast cancer survivors with associated significant health-related issues. Studies have shown that hot flashes are among the most severe and frequent symptoms experienced by over two-thirds of women during the menopause transition as function of the ovaries begins to decline with reduced production of estrogen. Having the ovaries surgically removed can lead to similar and even more severe hot flashes. Hot flashes among breast cancer survivors is as high as 90% due to several reasons including chemotherapy altering the function of the ovaries, surgical removal of the ovaries, or medications utilized to prevent cancer recurrence. Furthermore, hot flashes can be severe, causing anxiety and other emotional alterations, sleep disturbances, and interference with family, work, and social activities, all of which can negatively affect quality of life.

For the millions of women currently experiencing distressing hot flashes, there is a wide array of treatments. As with the management of most medical disorders, one size does not fit all as women may vary in their personal preferences, response to various treatments, and side effects and risks. While estrogen therapy, alone or in combination with progesterone, is an FDA-approved and very effective treatment option for hot flashes, there are rare associated risks for some women, making many fearful to use such products and causing reluctance by many health care providers to prescribe estrogen products. Unfortunately, many women continue to "put up" with life-altering hot flashes because they are not aware that other effective treatment options exist.

As a practicing obstetrics and gynecology (OB/GYN) physician, medical school professor, and researcher, I am pleased to recommend this book on hypnosis relaxation therapy, *Relief from Hot Flashes: The Natural, Drug-Free Program to Reduce Hot Flashes, Improve*

Sleep, and Ease Stress as an effective treatment option for women experiencing distressing hot flashes and night sweats. What you hold in your hands is a book that not only provides the most up-to-date information on hot flashes, but also provides a detailed tool for reducing hot flashes. All the forms needed for monitoring symptoms along with the audio recordings of actual hypnotic relaxation therapy sessions are included.

Dr. Gary Elkins' clinical practice and many years of research have resulted in the development of a five-week program that can significantly reduce hot flashes and associated symptoms such as stress and disrupted sleep that can occur during menopause. Women who have used this program have achieved clinically significant relief from hot flashes, improved sleep, and reductions in feelings of anxiety and depression. Dr. Elkins' methods of hypnotic relaxation have been scientifically proven to reduce hot flashes by up to 70% to 80% for most women. However, until now the program was not readily available outside of Dr. Elkins' practice. I was very pleased to see the publication of this book because it makes this program easily accessible to women who want a choice and who wish to learn this method.

This is a very useful and empowering book. Women who follow Dr. Elkins' step-by-step outlined approach have not only personally taken control of their hot flashes, but also improved their emotional well-being and quality of life. I highly recommend this book as a proven treatment option for women with distressing hot flashes!

Patricia J. Sulak, MD.
Founder, *Living Well Aware*
Dudley P. Baker Endowed Professor of
Research and Education in Obstetrics and Gynecology,
Texas A&M University College of Medicine
Medical Director, Division of Research,
Department of Obstetrics and Gynecology
Baylor Scott & White Health

Preface

My interest in mind–body medicine and hypnotic relaxation therapy began while I was completing my doctoral degree at Texas A&M University and my clinical internship at Wilford Hall USAF Medical Center in San Antonio, Texas. In 1981, while completing my internship, I was fortunate to attend a workshop on the use of clinical hypnosis and hypnotic relaxation therapy in health care presented by Dr. Harold Crasilneck. Dr. Crasilneck was a leading expert in the field and I learned a great deal from him. I was seeing many patients with problems ranging from chronic pain to difficulty with sleep and stress. As I began to apply these methods in my clinical work, I was impressed with the benefits from teaching patients how to use relaxation, mental imagery, and the connection between the mind and the body. However, at that time I did not yet know of the potential of hypnotic relaxation therapy to help women with hot flashes and menopausal symptoms—that discovery came much later.

After completion of my doctoral studies at Texas A&M University, I was licensed as a psychologist and continued my work as a clinical health psychologist at Scott and White Clinic and Hospital in Temple, Texas. Scott and White Clinic is a major medical center in Central Texas with over 550 physicians representing virtually every medical specialty. It is also the clinical campus for the Texas A&M University Medical School. This was the ideal environment for me to further develop my interests in mind–body medicine and hypnotic relaxation therapy because many patients with medical problems can benefit from interventions such as relaxation therapy, learning positive health behaviors, and behavioral therapies. I was able to establish a behavioral medicine service and Mind–Body Medicine Research Laboratory and I continued to learn from my patients and the use of these types of therapies.

At the same time, my expertise in hypnotic relaxation therapy continued to develop. I became the chair of the regional workshop programs for the American Society of Clinical Hypnosis and over the years taught literally hundreds of workshops and program nationally and internationally. In 1996, I was elected President of the American Society of Clinical Hypnosis and co-authored an important publication, *Standards of Training in Clinical Hypnosis*, for health care professionals. In addition, I was later elected to serve as the President of the American Board of Psychological Hypnosis and received board certification from the American Board of Professional Psychology in Clinical Health Psychology. My research program began to thrive and I obtained several grants to study the effect of hypnotic relaxation for improving the quality of life of cancer patients and in pain management. I published numerous journal articles as a result. All of these experiences were very gratifying and enabled me to eventually develop a safe and effective mind–body therapy for hot flashes among breast cancer survivors and postmenopausal women.

It was in 2003 that my focus began to shift to the study of hot flashes, and it continues to be the primary focus of my work. During that year, while I was conducting a study of hypnotic relaxation for pain management among cancer patients, the National Institutes of Health (NIH) released the initial results from a major study, the Women's Health Initiative Study. The study is described in more detail later in this book; however, the essential finding from this large study of over 16,000 postmenopausal women was that the hormone therapy that had been used to treat hot flashes is associated with an increased risk of breast cancer and cardiovascular disease. It became apparent that there was a pressing need to find an effective *nonhormonal* treatment for hot flashes.

One of the oncologists that I was working with at that time, Dr. Robyn Young, suggested to me that I might try hypnotic relaxation therapy with one of her patients who was experiencing severe hot flashes as a side effect of her treatment for breast cancer. I readily agreed to try and the patient was scheduled for several sessions with me. To her delight and frankly, to Dr. Young's surprise, the patient began to experience a marked reduction in her hot flashes. In fact, by the end of treatment she was no longer having any night sweats and only an occasional mild hot flash during the day. We decided this was something that needed to be understood and further studied.

I was then able to acquire an initial grant from the National Cancer Institute to do a pilot study of hypnotic relaxation therapy for hot flashes among breast cancer survivors. I was joined by Dr. Joel Marcus as a postdoctoral fellow (who is now Director of the Psychosocial Oncology Service at Oschner Clinic in New Orleans) and we completed a study of 60 breast cancer survivors with hot flashes. Half of them were randomized to receive hypnotic relaxation therapy and half were on a wait-list to receive the treatment later. By the end of the study, women who received hypnotic relaxation therapy had reduced their hot flashes by almost 70% on average.

While we were pleased with these findings, more work needed to be done. While it appeared that a mind–body therapy could significantly reduce hot flashes, we did not yet know if the intervention would work as well with healthy postmenopausal women. Also, more study was needed to find out if the reduction in hot flashes could be verified by physiological monitoring and if the benefit could be maintained even after the women stopped attending sessions.

By this time I had accepted a position at Baylor University as a Professor and Director of the Clinical Psychology Program. Baylor University provided me with the support and facilities to establish a fully functioning Mind–Body Medicine Research Laboratory, and with funding from the National Center for Complementary and Alternative Medicine of the NIH, I set out to conduct a large randomized clinical trial to answer these important questions.

The next study was conducted over five years and involved postmenopausal women who were experiencing moderate to severe hot flashes. The details of this groundbreaking study are provided in this book. The study was the first to establish that hypnotic relaxation therapy could reduce hot flashes as measured by both self-report and physiological recordings. By the end of the study we were able to show that the women's hot flashes had been reduced by 80% on average.

The study also showed additional benefits including improved sleep, reduced stress, and better quality of life. At this point, we were establishing the efficacy of this treatment. It is something women can learn to do and report to be pleasant and relaxing. The treatment was developed to provide five sessions over about five weeks using finely developed hypnotic relaxation inductions, audio recordings of sessions, training in self-hypnosis, and use of specialized rating scales to measure hot flashes. However, it was still not very widely available to women due to the need for women to travel to Baylor University in Waco, Texas, in order to receive the treatment program.

To meet this need, the present book, *Relief from Hot Flashes: The Natural, Drug-Free Program to Reduce Hot Flashes, Improve Sleep, and Ease Stress* was written. The book, for the first time, provides the same information and step-by-step guidance that women in the previous studies at the Mind–Body Medicine Research Laboratory at Baylor University received. Including access to five audio sessions to help guide you through the daily practice of hypnotic relaxation therapy and the same assessment forms used in the study (available at www.demoshealth.com/store/elkins-relief-from-hot-flashes-supplements), *Relief from Hot Flashes* is designed to provide all of the information needed to achieve positive results, reduce hot flashes, and learn the potential of hypnotic relaxation therapy and the mind–body connection. In using this program, it is important to follow all of the steps in the order they are presented.

The methods presented in *Relief from Hot Flashes* have helped many women to reduce their hot flashes, sleep better, and reduce stress; and it can help you too!

Gary Elkins, PhD, ABPP, ABPH
Director, Mind–Body Medicine Research Laboratory
Baylor University

Acknowledgments

This book is the result of years of clinical research in the Mind–Body Medicine Research Laboratory (MBMRL) and practice with hundreds of women with hot flashes. I have been fortunate to be blessed with excellent colleagues, students, and fellow researchers in the quest to identify an effective mind–body treatment for symptoms women experience during the menopause transition.

I would like to acknowledge the funding and support I have received from the National Center for Complementary and Alternative Medicine (NCCAM) and from the National Cancer Institute (NCI) of the NIH. My work and the MBMRL have been continually supported by NCCAM and NCI for the past 10 years and this has made it possible to develop the knowledge presented in this book. While the work is my own and does not and should not be interpreted as representing the NIH, the support has been invaluable.

I am grateful for the support I have received from Baylor University and specifically from Dr. Jaime Diaz-Granados, Chair of the Department of Psychology and Neuroscience who has provided encouragement, time, and the resources needed.

I want to express my gratitude to Vicki Patterson, B.A., who is the Clinical Research Coordinator in the MBMRL at Baylor University. Vicki assisted me not only with all aspects of my research into hot flashes, but also in review of multiple drafts of this manuscript and revisions, scales, and references.

I want to recognize the immense contributions of the many colleagues, students and post-doctoral fellows who have been instrumental in this process: Joel Marcus, PsyD; Jeff Bates, MD; Christopher Ruud, MD; Jacqueline Dove, PhD; Jennifer Bunn, PhD; Cassie Kendrick, PsyD; Lauren Koep, PsyD; William Fisher, PhD;

Aimee Johnson, MA; Jim Sliwinski, MA; Debra Barton, RN, PhD; Janet Carpenter, RN, PhD; Timothy Keith, PhD; Vered Stearns, MD; Robyn Young, MD; Carl Chakmakjian, MD; Carlos Encarnacion, MD; Catherine Stoney, PhD; and Lee Alekel, PhD.

I want to express my gratitude to Julia Pastore, Executive Editor at Demos Health Publishing, for her guidance and support in the development of this book.

Finally, I want to thank my loving wife and life partner, Guillerma Gamez Elkins for her encouragement and support. In addition to making sure I had the time needed, she helped me keep my personal balance while I was devoting the many hours to research and writing, guided me in better understanding women's health care needs, and read and re-read and edited the many drafts of this book.

Thank you all!

Relief from Hot Flashes

UNDERSTANDING HOT FLASHES

Chapter 1

How This Book Will Help You

The purpose of this book is to provide you with all of the information and resources needed to achieve relief from hot flashes. A step-by-step approach is used to introduce a proven program of hypnotic relaxation therapy for reducing hot flashes and improving health. You may be tempted to skip ahead, but reading and using the forms and audio files in the order they are presented will help you get the best results. The overall program takes about five weeks to complete. There are several audio files that accompany this book and you will need these to learn how to control your hot flashes. Research on the program is discussed to help you understand how and why it works. Knowing about this research may also be helpful to you if you want to discuss the program with your doctor.

Before we get to the "nuts and bolts" of hot flashes, ask yourself if you can relate to any of the following statements.

"Every night I go to sleep with a fan blowing air on me, but I still wake up several times soaking with sweat and have trouble going back to sleep."

"I feel embarrassed at work. I'm a teacher and the kids laugh when I blush red and start perspiring."

"I turn the air conditioner down, but my husband keeps turning it back up. We have been sleeping in different rooms because I keep throwing the covers off and then pulling them back on."

"I get so nervous when I start having hot flashes; sometimes they come every 30 minutes; I know I get irritable."

If you have hot flashes, you probably have been told different things. You may have been told that you will just have to suffer through them or that they will just "go away." The fact is that hot flashes can last for months or years; some women continue to have them into their 80s! Various remedies may have been suggested to you, most of which probably did not work all that well. You may have heard about the risks associated with hormone therapy and have concerns about taking pharmaceutical estrogen. You would like to know about alternatives to hormone replacement therapy.

Hot flashes are among the most common symptoms women experience during the menopausal transition and almost all women have hot flashes at some time in their lives. Millions of women in the United States have hot flashes and of those, about 20% have severe hot flashes resulting in distress and interference with daily activities. However, not everyone experiences hot flashes in the same way. For some women hot flashes occur as unwelcome sensations of warmth that are simply annoying and bothersome. For others, they may be intense and frequent. For many women, hot flashes occur as waves of heat, flushing, rapid heartbeat, and being drenched in sweat almost hourly. Further, hot flashes can occur both during the day *and* night. When they occur during sleep they are called "night sweats" and result in sleep being disrupted multiple times during the night. Other symptoms associated with hot flashes include fatigue, irritability, anxiety, and, for some, depression. When hot flashes are frequent they can have negative consequences that affect virtually every aspect of a woman's life—social, psychological, and

> Hot flashes are among the most common symptoms women experience during the menopausal transition and almost all women have hot flashes at some time in their lives.

health. This is reflected in the statements above, made to me by women as they described their hot flashes.

It is important to know that hot flashes are physiological events that occur with the onset of menopause when estrogen levels decline. Many women are interested in finding safe and effective ways to reduce hot flashes. Research has shown that there is an alternative to the use of drugs and hormones alone. That alternative is a mind–body therapy that involves learning the techniques of hypnotic relaxation therapy, mental imagery, and the practice of self-hypnosis.

Hypnotic relaxation therapy for hot flashes is something you learn to do; it is not something that is done to you. It requires active participation.

Before discussing the program, I would like to acknowledge that you may be optimistic or skeptical or somewhere in between. If you have had some previous positive experience with hypnotic relaxation, then you may have a head start as you already have some knowledge that will likely be of benefit.

If you are skeptical, then I would say that is understandable. This is a new and innovative program and you are among the first to learn it. By reading this book you will gain a lot of knowledge and become informed about hypnotic relaxation therapy, both how to do it and what the research has shown. However, most of us are convinced by our own experience. As you follow the steps outlined here and your hot flashes begin to decrease, you will progressively develop the confidence you need.

If you are somewhere in between, then please keep in mind that the most important thing is to follow the steps provided in this book and maintain consistent practice. By keeping an open mind, you will be able to "get into" the program and achieve your goals.

Hypnotic relaxation therapy for hot flashes is something you learn to do; it is not something that is done to you (like taking a pill). It requires active participation. Therefore, you will be provided the tools to take control and be actively involved in your own health care.

HOW TO USE THIS BOOK

I believe that knowledge is necessary for sound decision making and learning a new skill. This book is organized to provide you with the knowledge needed to develop the skills necessary to significantly reduce your hot flashes.

To begin, I'll present the research in support of this program so that you will have a good understanding of the evidence behind hypnotic relaxation therapy. I'll also discuss the causes of hot flashes along with the pros and cons of hormone replacement therapy and alternatives.

Next, in "First Things First," you will learn how to record your hot flashes and determine the frequency and severity with which they occur. This will give you the information you need to track your progress. You will also learn how to identify any triggers for hot flashes and to rate your sleep and mood.

After you have kept a diary of the frequency and severity of your hot flashes for at least a week, you will be ready to start the five- week program outlined in the next section, "Hypnotic Relaxation Therapy: The Solution for Hot Flashes." You will learn how to use the audio files that accompany this book and begin practicing the techniques of hypnotic relaxation to reduce your hot flashes. It is very important that you use the audio recordings exactly as indicated. You should only use the audio recordings when you can sit or lie down for about 30 to 45 minutes and be undisturbed. You should never use the audio recordings when you are driving a car or engaging in *any* other activity. You will also learn how to use self-hypnosis.

As you monitor your progress you will be able to see how your hot flashes become less frequent, and you will also likely notice that they are beginning to shift toward becoming less severe or intense. After completing the hypnotic relaxation program for five weeks

To access the audio recordings and all of the tracking and assessment forms mentioned in the book, visit www .demoshealth.com/store/elkins-relief-from-hot-flashes-supplements you will be provided with forms and guidance that will help you to assess your progress.

Finally, I hope the insights and experiences of the three women who have completed this program, included in the Afterword, will provide assurance, encouragement, and motivation.

EVIDENCE THIS PROGRAM WILL WORK FOR YOU

In my clinical practice, I have been able to work with several hundred women who were referred to me for management of hot flashes and associated symptoms. Over the years of practice, I have been able to refine the hypnotic relaxation therapy program to be most efficient in the control of hot flashes. In this regard, most women have been able to learn the methods and effectively reduce their hot flashes. In addition, there is considerable evidence that the program reduces hot flashes among women who are postmenopause or who have hot flashes as a result of treatment for breast cancer. The research has been consistent and provides evidence of the effectiveness of the program.

Research conducted at the Mind–Body Medicine Research Laboratory at Baylor University demonstrated that women who used the hypnotic relaxation therapy program were able to reduce their hot flashes to a very high degree and in some cases eliminate them altogether. In the latest study, women recorded their hot flashes at the beginning of the study, while receiving treatment, and at a follow-up three months later. In addition, the women wore special monitors that recorded sweating associated with hot flashes. The reduction in hot flashes

> Women who used the hypnotic relaxation therapy program were able to reduce their hot flashes by 80% on average.

was apparent in both self-reports and by physiological monitoring. At the end of the study, women who used hypnotic relaxation had a reduction in hot flashes of 80% on average. Treatment satisfaction was very high for the women who received hypnotic relaxation therapy with a rating of about "9" on a 0 to 10 scale (with "10" representing *completely satisfied*). The study was supported by the National Center for Complementary and Alternative Medicine (NCCAM), a division of the National Institutes of Health (NIH); however, I want to acknowledge that the opinions are solely the responsibility of the author and do not necessarily represent the views of the NIH.

In this book, you will receive the same materials, diaries, audio recordings, and other materials that were available to the women in the Baylor study. Just as the program has worked for them, it can work for you.

YOU MAY BE SURPRISED AT HOW QUICKLY HOT FLASHES DECREASE

The idea that a mind–body therapy such as the daily practice of hypnotic relaxation and mental imagery can significantly reduce hot flashes may be a new concept to you. Through your own experience and practice you will discover how it works for you personally. It is my belief that you may be surprised at how quickly your hot flashes decrease. For many women the reduction in the number of hot flashes is quite apparent after the first or second week of daily practice. The results from a study I published in the *International Journal of Clinical and Experimental Hypnosis* are shown in the following chart.

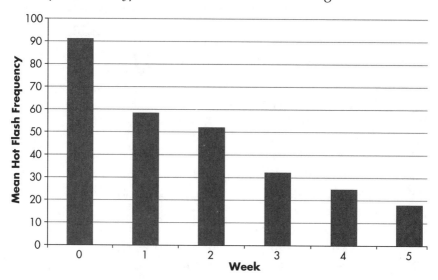

Average frequency of hot flashes by weeks in program.

The study of postmenopausal women who completed the *Relief from Hot Flashes* program indicated a reduction in the frequency of hot flashes of: **30% after week 1; 40% after week 2; 60% after week 3; 65% after week 4; and 78% after week 5 of practice!** As you can see, the improvement can occur within weeks; however, *continued practice is required* to maintain the progress.

BETTER SLEEP CAN BE ACHIEVED

Good sleep is important for your overall quality of life. However, it has been found that sleep is affected by the onset of menopause and hot flashes. In fact, about 40% to 60% of all postmenopausal women and 80% of women with severe hot flashes report poor sleep. Better sleep can be achieved with this program.

In the study mentioned above, over 180 women with hot flashes were randomized to receive either the hypnotic relaxation program or structured attention counseling sessions. In that study, the women recorded their hot flashes, and those randomized to the hypnotic relaxation program were able to reduce hot flashes by about 80% on average. The women also recorded the quality of their sleep before and after using the hypnotic relaxation audio recordings. The results are shown on the following page. You can see that hypnotic relaxation improved their sleep, with overall self-reported sleep quality improved by about 70%. The findings also indicated that the women reported reduced sleep latency (the length of time that it takes to transition from full wakefulness to sleep). For the women who practiced hypnotic relaxation, sleep latency improved by 50% at 12-week

> Good sleep is important for your overall quality of life. Better sleep can be achieved with this program.

follow-up. At baseline, postmenopausal women in the study reported an average of 41 minutes to fall asleep. However, after using hypnotic relaxation and listening to the audio recordings they reported, on average, 19 minutes to fall asleep. Another indicator of good sleep is sleep duration (the total hours slept). For the women who practiced hypnotic relaxation, sleep duration improved by 49% at 12-week follow-up. This suggests that the women who used hypnotic relaxation were getting, on average, approximately seven to eight hours of good sleep at the end of the study. The results also indicated that postmenopausal women who used hypnotic relaxation for hot flashes reported a decrease in use of sleep medication with a change of 50%.

CHANGES IN SLEEP QUALITY WITH HYPNOTIC RELAXATION

MEASURE OF SLEEP	PERCENTAGE IMPROVEMENT IN SLEEP
SLEEP QUALITY	
6 wk	68.93%
12 wk	70.38%
SLEEP LATENCY	
6 wk	41.53%
12 wk	51.28%
SLEEP DURATION	
6 wk	44.44%
12 wk	46.91%
USE OF SLEEP MEDICATION	
6 wk	43.24%
12 wk	48.65%

In the studies noted above, overall sleep quality improved significantly with the hypnotic relaxation intervention. Women who reported only five to six hours of sleep each night at baseline, experienced improved sleep duration to seven to eight hours by their 12-week follow-up appointment. In addition, women reported being able to go to sleep more quickly when using the audio recordings that are included as a part of this program, as well as reduce their use of sleep medication.

YOU WILL LEARN TO FEEL LESS STRESS

As you begin to practice hypnotic relaxation you will likely find that you are able to feel more relaxed while listening to the audio recordings. As relaxation is achieved, there are physiological changes that occur such as decreased muscle tension, lowered heart rate, and changes in blood pressure. You are also likely to notice that you feel calmer while using the audio recordings as instructed in this book. With daily practice, this sense of calmness can last longer and longer. Many women report that they feel calmer in their daily life—things do not bother them as much, and they feel better able to cope with stress. This is a benefit I feel certain you will appreciate beyond the reduction in hot flashes!

INDIVIDUAL PREFERENCES MATTER

As you begin to learn the methods outlined in this book, the audio recordings will guide you through general hypnotic suggestions that have been shown to be "tried and true" to reduce hot flashes. However, you will very likely find that you have some preferences for mental imagery that work best for you. These individual preferences matter, and I will show you how to use them to help you progress toward the benefits more quickly. For example, some women prefer the mental imagery of walking down a mountain path with snow all around, while others may prefer imagery of sitting near a lake. In studies of hypnotic relaxation therapy for hot flashes, the imagery chosen by most women included mountains, water, air/wind, snow, and trees/leaves. Of these, the most widely used was water associated with coolness (29.5%). The use of imagery may be a significant contributor to the reduction of hot flashes and *individualized imagery* has been shown in previous research to be a beneficial part of treatment effectiveness.

OTHER SYMPTOMS OF MENOPAUSE

There are three stages of the menopausal transition that women experience, and there are symptoms that occur during each stage.

Perimenopause refers to the time when estrogen levels begin to decline and can last for several years before the onset of natural menopause. During perimenopause women begin to experience hot flashes, irregular menstrual periods, vaginal dryness, and sleep disturbance. There can also be mood swings during this transition period.

Menopause is defined as the ending of menstrual periods. Most women begin menopause between the ages of 40 and 58. The average age for the onset of natural menopause is 51; however, women who smoke may go into menopause a couple of years earlier. Hot flashes occur more frequently during menopause, as do sleep problems.

Postmenopause is the time after menopause, which may be several years. In fact, most women spend about a third of their life in postmenopause. Menstrual periods completely stop and hot flashes are the most common problem. In addition, sleep complaints continue for many women. Also, changes in memory and concentration may occur during the menopausal transition. Sexual desire may decline, although factors other than the change in estrogen can contribute to issues related to sexuality and romantic relationships. Some women experience weight gain, and skin changes occur because there is a loss of collagen and elasticity. Energy or mood may be varied with the abrupt alteration in estrogen.

The hypnotic relaxation program can help you with many of these symptoms.

WHAT TO TELL YOUR FAMILY AND COWORKERS

If you are going through menopause, it is usually best to let your family know of any symptoms that you are experiencing and how you are dealing with them. It can be especially helpful to let your family, friends, or coworkers know about your symptoms if you are having hot flashes or increased stress.

Once you begin recording your hot flashes and using the methods of hypnotic relaxation therapy provided here, you will want to let people in your life know that you are using a mind–body therapy and that you need time to practice these methods. You will need about 30 minutes one or more times a day to practice hypnotic relaxation. During these times, you should be in a quiet place where you will not be disturbed.

YOU MAY BE TAKING MEDICATION FOR HOT FLASHES

Antidepressant medication is sometimes prescribed for hot flashes. If you have been taking medication (such as antidepressants) for hot flashes, it will not affect your use of this program. The hypnotic relaxation program will work regardless of whether or not you are taking such medications. It is your personal preference; however, it may be reassuring to know that the women in the studies of this program were all able to discontinue other treatments for hot flashes. If you are taking medications and consider stopping them, you should certainly discuss it with your physician before making any changes.

TALK TO YOUR DOCTOR

You should talk to your doctor about all aspects of your health care as he or she can provide answers to your questions about menopause and hot flashes. Your personal health care provider is the best person to guide you in regard to decisions about your health. Always contact your doctor if you notice any physical changes or concerns. This book can help you with hot flashes; however, it is not a replacement, in any way, for your health care provider. You should also have regular check-ups that may identify health conditions and/or concerns, and then discuss these issues with your doctor.

❋

In summary, this book will help you in many ways! You will gain knowledge about the life stages of menopause, hot flashes, and related symptoms. You will be given tips on stress management, how to improve your sleep, and when to seek advice from your doctor. But the most valuable tools you will likely take from this book are the skills that will help you to significantly reduce your hot flashes and to work toward gaining control of and being actively involved in your own overall health care.

Chapter 2

What Causes Hot Flashes?

Hot flashes have a physical cause; they occur most often in women before, during, and after menopause, and can continue for years. The hormonal changes that occur during this time, including lower levels of estrogen, are associated with the onset of hot flashes. They are not caused by a woman's mood, attitude, or emotions. During a hot flash there is an abrupt change in core body temperature that causes sweating. In this chapter we will review what happens during a hot flash, the physiology and psychology of hot flashes, as well as the role of other factors such as weather, anxiety, tension, and stress. This information will be helpful to you as you learn to use the hypnotic relaxation program to reduce hot flashes.

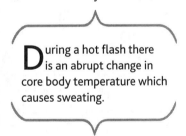

During a hot flash there is an abrupt change in core body temperature which causes sweating.

WHAT HAPPENS DURING A HOT FLASH

A hot flash is an event in which there is a sudden feeling of heat and perspiration. Some women notice an "aura" just moments before the onset of a hot flash. These auras vary and have been described in different ways.

"I get a feeling of light-headedness or dizziness, and within a few seconds, I can feel the flush starting on my neck and chest."

"Most times right before a hot flash, I feel a rush of coolness and nausea, like something being poured over my head and running down over my body."

"I always feel very anxious, sort of panicky, then after a little bit, I start feeling a tingling sensation on my scalp; then the sweating starts and moves down over my face, neck and chest."

Skin temperature rises rapidly as blood rushes to the face and a wave of heat sensation spreads over the upper body and chest. Heart rate increases as the face becomes flushed. Profuse sweating is followed by evaporation from those areas, leading to a decrease in body temperature and a chilled feeling as the hot flash passes.

A hot flash can last for as little as a few seconds or as long as 15 minutes. They can occur throughout the day, and some women report having them as often as every 30 to 60 minutes. Because hot flashes follow a well-defined pattern of dilation of the blood vessels near the skin and a sudden outpouring of sweat, they can be measured objectively. In a recent clinical study women with hot flashes were asked to wear a sternal skin conductance device that measures hot flashes. The device, called a "Biolog®," measures the frequency of hot flashes to record each occurrence. The chart on the facing page illustrates the frequency and the course of hot flashes during a day in a 52-year old woman.

The spikes indicate a hot flash and their objective measurement. This woman was having about 15 hot flashes per day before she began using the hypnotic relaxation.

Small changes in temperature, emotions, and even certain foods can trigger a hot flash. Additional factors that can contribute to hot flashes are smoking and the use of alcohol. In a sense, the onset of a hot flash is an attempt to cool the body. The brain perceives heat (although no heat is present) and that prompts a physiological chain reaction which ultimately leads to sweating.

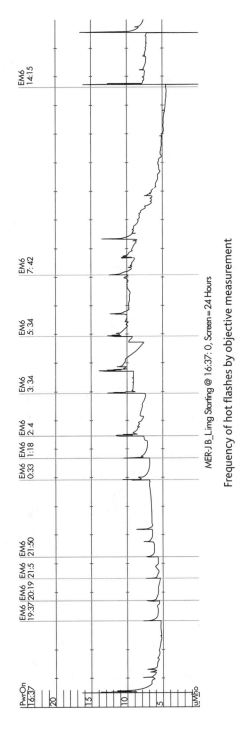

MER-J B_Limg Starting @ 16:37: 0, Screen = 24 Hours

Frequency of hot flashes by objective measurement

This chain reaction is similar to what happens with the *stress response*. The sympathetic nervous system goes into overdrive; vasodilation of the vessels in the skin occurs; and there is an overall arousal of stress and tension.

SEVERITY

The "severity" of a hot flash refers to how severely a woman experiences the event. Research has shown that women can reliably distinguish between a mild, moderate, severe, or very severe hot flash. When hot flashes are severe or very severe they can interfere with daily activities and may be accompanied by feelings of panic or loss of control.

> When hot flashes are severe or very severe they can interfere with daily activities and may be accompanied by feelings of panic or loss of control.

PHYSIOLOGY OF HOT FLASHES

The *hypothalamus* is an area of the brain that regulates body temperature and recent evidence suggests that the hypothalamus plays an important role in the physiology of hot flashes. It is likely that the changes in hormone levels affect the hypothalamus's ability to perceive and regulate temperature.

The *"neutral zone"* refers to a state in which we feel comfortable (i.e., neither too hot nor too cold). It may be that prior to perimenopause you were working outdoors on a hot summer day and experienced a "hot flash"—sweating, flushing, redness. The hypothalamus perceives that the body has become overheated and attempts to regulate the body's temperature by initiating these physiological reactions. This is explained by the neutral zone. Prior to a woman's normal hormonal changes that begin in perimenopause, the neutral zone is wide, and it takes a significant event to trigger a hot flash (i.e., extreme temperature or stress). However, as a woman begins the menopausal transition, the "neutral zone" narrows, meaning

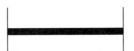

NARROW neutral zone = MORE hot flashes

WIDE neutral zone = FEWER hot flashes

that slight changes in temperature can trigger a hot flash. Hypnotic relaxation therapy works to widen the neutral zone, and *as the neutral zone becomes wider, hot flashes decrease.* These illustrations show the difference between a narrow and a wide neutral zone.

With this visual of your *neutral zone,* it is my goal to help you imagine your neutral zone widening as your hot flashes decrease. Over time, as the neutral zone widens, hot flashes become less and less frequent!

PSYCHOLOGY OF HOT FLASHES

When hot flashes are frequent they can be embarrassing, cause strain at work, and affect social relationships. In addition, hot flashes can disrupt sleep, which can result in chronic feelings of fatigue and lack of energy. It is important for you to be aware of these psychological aspects of hot flashes, and they should be addressed in order to help you feel better and achieve success as you work to minimize their frequency and severity.

For some women, the heat associated with hot flashes causes them to want to avoid close physical contact or to avoid intimacy as they fear this may trigger a hot flash. This avoidance can cause tension in marital and intimate relationships and contribute to a depressed mood. For most of us, our personal relationships and mood are among the most important aspects of our lives. It is no small statement to acknowledge that the psychology of hot flashes is just as important as the physiology.

ANXIETY, STRESS, AND HOT FLASHES

While anxiety and stress do not cause hot flashes, they can certainly make them worse! Often, women report that their hot flashes become worse during times of stress. For example, one of my patients, Donna,[*] reported that she could anticipate having more hot flashes while she was at work than at any other time. She was employed in a highly stressful job in the customer service department for a telephone and cable television company. She stated that there were days when she felt overwhelmed due to the amount of phone calls that she had to process, often with irate customers, and her tendency to be overly critical of herself. As she learned to take more time for herself and learned better ways of coping with stress, she noticed she was better able to control her hot flashes and to remain calmer. Stress management can be an important part of gaining relief from hot flashes.

> While anxiety and stress do not cause hot flashes, they can certainly make them worse!

CAN MEN HAVE HOT FLASHES?

Yes, men can have hot flashes just as women do. The reasons men have hot flashes are, of course, not related to estrogen. Rather, hot flashes occur in men who either have a history of prostate cancer or another disorder causing an androgen (male hormone testosterone) deficiency. Up to 80% of all prostate cancer survivors experience hot flashes, and about 50% of those experience them as severe and needing treatment. Further, when men have hot flashes due to prostate cancer, the hot flashes tend to be more frequent and continue for a longer period of

---

[*] Note: Throughout this book all names and identifying characteristics of case studies have been changed to protect individuals' privacy.

time in comparison to those associated with menopause. Hot flashes have been cited as being one of the most distressing symptoms associated with prostate cancer treatment. While most of the research on hypnotic relaxation therapy for hot flashes has focused on women, either postmenopause or breast cancer survivors, it is very likely that hypnotic relaxation and the program included in this book will work as well for men as it does for women.

❋

Hot flashes have a physical cause; however, they can be affected by stress, sleep, and the environment. Understanding what causes hot flashes, how they are perceived, the physiological and psychological aspects of hot flashes, and what factors may contribute to making them worse is an important first step in moving forward to the treatment of this menopausal symptom. However, hot flashes are also often experienced by women after they receive treatment for breast cancer. If you are experiencing hot flashes as a result of breast cancer treatment, the next chapter explains how the *Relief from Hot Flashes* program can help you.

Chapter 3

Breast Cancer and Hot Flashes

Each year, over 200,000 women are diagnosed with breast cancer, and hot flashes are prevalent among these women. Breast cancer survivors who are postmenopausal at the time of diagnosis are likely to have hot flashes. In addition, the treatment for breast cancer often induces menopause and hot flashes in younger women. The methods of treatment such as chemotherapy, radiation, and surgical removal of ovaries can induce menopause in women who are not yet menopausal. It is generally recognized that hot flashes that are induced by breast cancer

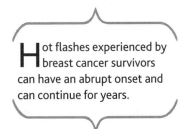

Hot flashes experienced by breast cancer survivors can have an abrupt onset and can continue for years.

treatment can be more intense and severe than those that occur through natural menopause. This is because estrogen production is abruptly stopped and the onset of hot flashes is very sudden. It is estimated that 51% to 81% of women with breast cancer experience hot flashes, and the hot flashes can last for years.

Most breast cancers are sensitive to estrogen, and following treatment medications may be prescribed that prevent estrogen production completely. This can lead to moderate to severe hot flashes and associated symptoms such as sleep disturbance, vaginal dryness, and changes in mood. The diagnosis of breast cancer can be very stressful, and this can affect hot flashes as well.

If you are a breast cancer survivor, the *Relief from Hot Flashes* program can help relieve hot flashes as well as help relieve stress.

CANCER TREATMENT AND HOT FLASHES

Following a diagnosis of breast cancer, there are a number of treatments that may be considered. These include intervention to reduce the size or remove cancer tissue. Other treatments are designed to reduce the production of estrogen.

Surgery

There are two types of surgical intervention that are designed to remove tumor tissue: lumpectomy and mastectomy. Lumpectomy is more conservative and removes only the breast tumor and an amount of surrounding tissue. This is a procedure that is considered for many breast cancers and can have a positive cosmetic result (as breast tissue is preserved) and is less traumatic than mastectomy. However, it can have some risk of local recurrence. Mastectomy involves the removal of most or all breast tissue and can also involve removal of the muscles in the chest wall (called radical mastectomy). Surgery can be an effective treatment that can affect body image as well as being stressful.

Chemotherapy

Chemotherapy is often used in combination with surgery or radiation therapy. It involves the use of drugs that are designed to reduce cancer cells. Chemotherapy can have side effects such as nausea, fatigue, hair loss, pain, and decreased immunity. However, these symptoms usually resolve when chemotherapy is discontinued.

Radiation Therapy

Radiation therapy can be effective in shrinking tumors and is used to prevent local recurrence of cancer. It can have side effects similar to chemotherapy such as fatigue. However, the benefits can include improved overall treatment.

Tamoxifen and Raloxifene

After treatment for breast cancer, drugs known as selective estrogen-receptor modulators (SERMs) may be prescribed. Two such drugs, tamoxifen (Nolvadex®) and raloxifene (Evista®), are often recommended for breast cancer prevention. These drugs shut down the production of estrogen and may be taken for approximately five years. Women at risk for breast cancer recurrence should discuss the risks and benefits with their physician. The use of tamoxifen or raloxifene usually results in hot flashes. Studies show that hot flashes are very prevalent (78%) among breast cancer survivors who receive tamoxifen medication. Further, 90% of premenopausal women with a history of breast cancer who receive both chemotherapy and a SERM therapy such as tamoxifen have hot flashes and associated symptoms. For some of these women the hot flashes can be severe.

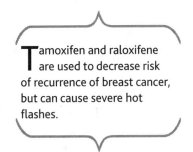

Tamoxifen and raloxifene are used to decrease risk of recurrence of breast cancer, but can cause severe hot flashes.

Aromatase Inhibitors

Aromatase inhibitors are another class of drugs used in the treatment of breast cancer in post-menopausal women. Aromatase inhibitors are a newer class of drug that work differently from tamoxifen and raloxifene. Instead of blocking estrogen receptors, they stop an enzyme (i.e. *aromatase*) from converting different hormones in the woman's body into estrogen. This lowers estrogen levels and thereby lowers the risk of recurrence of estrogen-receptor-positive breast cancer. Aromatase inhibitors include Aromasin® (exemestane),

Femara® (letrozole), and Arimidex® (anastrozole) and are most likely to be used in post-menopausal women and for treating advanced breast cancer. The short-term side effects are similar to tamoxifen and raloxifene and includes hot flashes and vaginal dryness (as estrogen levels decline markedly). Additional side effects can include joint pain or headaches. Also, aromatase inhibitors tend to speed up the rate of bone thinning and osteoporosis.

HYPNOTIC RELAXATION FOR HOT FLASHES AMONG BREAST CANCER SURVIVORS

The use of tamoxifen, raloxifene, or aromatase inhibitors can help prevent recurrence of breast cancer however, they suppress the production of estrogen and cause hot flashes. Fortunately, there is considerable evidence that the *Relief from Hot Flashes* program can very significantly reduce hot flashes that occur among breast cancer patients. Therefore, there is great interest in hypnotic relaxation because it has been shown to be safe and effective in reducing hot flashes among breast cancer survivors.

One of the first studies was a clinical trial using hypnotic relaxation therapy with breast cancer survivors having hot flashes. Breast cancer survivors with a history of moderate hot flashes were randomized to two "conditions": they received either the "hypnosis intervention" or a "control condition." Most of the women were taking either tamoxifen or raloxifene at the time of the study. Those in the "control condition" did not receive any treatment for hot flashes and were on a wait-list. Each patient in the "hypnosis intervention" received five weekly sessions of hypnotic relaxation therapy and engaged in daily practice of self-hypnosis with audio recordings. Throughout the clinical care, patients completed daily diaries of the frequency and severity of their hot flashes. Results indicated about a 70% decrease in hot flashes from baseline to end of treatment. The findings of this study are shown in the chart on the facing page.

The results showed that hot flashes could be well managed without hormone therapy or other drugs. All of the women in

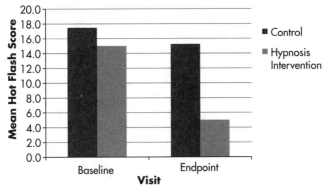

Hot flash scores for breast cancer survivors before and after receiving hypnosis intervention or control

this study had completed their treatment for breast cancer; however, some women experience hot flashes during treatment and it is helpful to consider the stage of breast cancer as this may affect stress and medical care.

BREAST CANCER DIAGNOSIS AND STAGE

Breast cancer is described by a staging system that takes into account the type, size, and location of tumor and whether the lymph nodes are involved. The earlier breast cancer is detected the more likely it is to be in an earlier stage, and thus the better prognosis will usually be with treatment.

Stage 0

Stage 0 is carcinoma in situ or Paget's disease of the nipple. It may be a slow-growing condition that can be treated with surgery and radiation.

Stage I

Stage I is a breast tumor that is 2 centimeters or less and has no lymph node involvement or metastases.

Stage IIA

Stage IIA can be used to describe two different conditions. It may be the same as stage 0 or stage 1, but with the involvement of lymph node(s) under the arm. Stage IIA can also refer to a tumor between 2 centimeters and 5 centimeters with no lymph node involvement.

Identification of the stage of breast cancer can help with treatment decisions and understanding the stresses of diagnosis.

Stage IIB

Stage IIB can also refer to two different conditions. It can refer to a tumor between 2 centimeters and 5 centimeters, with underarm lymph node involvement, or it can refer to a tumor of a size greater than 5 centimeters without lymph node involvement.

Stage IIIA

Stage IIIA can identify a tumor up to 5 centimeters in size with underarm lymph node involvement. However, there are not distant metastases and the tumor does not extend back to the chest wall.

Stage IIIB

Stage IIIB refers to a tumor that extends to the chest wall or skin. It can cause skin swelling or ulceration, or is inflammatory and involves underarm lymph nodes. It can also involve a tumor where mammary lymph nodes are involved, but there are no distant metastases.

Stage IV

State IV refers to breast cancer where there is spread to a distant metastatic site.

Identification of the breast cancer stage can aide in the selection of therapies for both short-term and long-term treatment. In general, earlier stages are likely to be more amenable to treatment.

In addition, breast cancer can have a significant impact on emotional well-being. Further, it can affect cognition, relationships, and self-esteem. Hypnotic relaxation methods can be helpful in coping with these factors as well as in reducing hot flashes.

EMOTIONAL, COGNITIVE, AND RELATIONAL IMPACT OF BREAST CANCER

Anxiety

Breast cancer is a very stressful life event that can cause distress and worry. In studies it has been shown that 80% of women with breast cancer report substantial distress, including fears, worries about recurrence, and financial concerns. In addition, the treatments for breast cancer, such as surgery and chemotherapy, provoke anxiety and concerns. For some women the anxiety may contribute to hot flashes, nausea, and a reduction in compliance with treatments that are recommended.

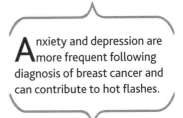

Anxiety and depression are more frequent following diagnosis of breast cancer and can contribute to hot flashes.

Risk for Depression

Undoubtedly, a diagnosis of breast cancer increases a woman's risk for developing depression. Factors that have been associated with increased levels of depression include the appraisal of threat, level of physical disability, cancer stage, and pre-existing history of depression. While most women experience some depression during treatment, the risk of becoming clinically depressed increases over time in dealing with breast cancer.

The most common type of clinical depression is major depression. This is a clinical diagnosis of depression in which the core symptoms are depressed mood and loss of interest or pleasure for most of the day and nearly every day. A major depression episode involves symptoms of severe depression that have continued for over two weeks or more. The symptoms of major depression are both physical and psychological, including continual depressed mood, markedly diminished interest in most activities, significant change in weight (weight loss when not dieting) due to changes in appetite, insomnia or hypersomnia, fatigue, feelings of worthlessness or hopelessness, indecisiveness, inability to concentrate, feelings of agitation, and thoughts of death or suicide (with or without a plan for self-harm).

This combination of depressive symptoms is a serious concern, and if you experience them you should discuss this with your doctor, pastor, friends, or family. If you have thoughts of suicide, then you should go to the hospital emergency room nearest to you without hesitation. There are therapies that can help a lot,

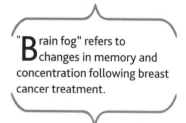

"Brain fog" refers to changes in memory and concentration following breast cancer treatment.

and just talking with a professional can relieve some of the burden and stress.

"Brain Fog" and Concentration

One of the cognitive effects of breast cancer treatments is on memory and concentration. This is a side effect of chemotherapy or radiation that sometimes is called "brain fog" because of the feeling of "being in a fog," in which memory is slower and the woman may feel distracted. It is important to recognize that these symptoms are real and that they are likely to resolve over time. There can also be stress associated with "brain fog" as it can make work more difficult, and the effect on memory causes worry for some women. Methods that reduce stress such as hypnotic relaxation therapy can have a positive effect on reducing "brain fog."

Relationships

Breast cancer can have a large impact on interpersonal relationships. The anxiety and medical demands associated with the diagnosis of breast cancer can cause the woman to withdraw from social activities at work, through her place of worship, or in the community. This can lead to a sense of isolation from others and contribute to the stress of breast cancer. In addition, the treatment for breast cancer, such as tamoxifen (Nolvadex) and raloxifene (Evista), can cause difficulty in sexual functioning. Further, hot flashes can interfere with intimate relationships due to a fear that the closeness of sexual activity may trigger hot flashes. Because of this, seeking support and effective coping can be important aspects of dealing with breast cancer. In this book, I will provide detailed information on how to reduce hot flashes with hypnotic relaxation and how this can also be helpful in managing stress. However, as discussed below, there are several other considerations in seeking support and coping with breast cancer that can be especially useful.

SUPPORT AND COPING WITH BREAST CANCER

Recognize Adjustment Issues

It is very important to recognize that feelings of stress and anxiety, changes in memory and concentration, and even the hot flashes that come with treatment for breast cancer are all normal. These adjustment issues are to be expected, and when they are recognized and acknowledged they can be best dealt with in an effective manner. By using the methods of hypnotic relaxation outlined in this book you will learn to relax, and as your hot flashes decrease you will find that you feel calmer and more in control.

Share Your Feelings

People who deny or hold their feelings inward tend to feel more stressed over time. It is important to seek emotional support from others. Communicating with others about your thoughts and feelings can include talking about the stress associated with breast cancer or the things that people generally talk about and are important in their lives. For most people this involves topics related to health as well as to family, friends, work, and relationships with others.

Remembering to share your feelings can be "powerful medicine" in coping with the stress of breast cancer.

Self-Care and Emotional Support

Along with emotional support is the necessity of self-care. Self-care involves taking time each day for reflection and relaxation. It can involve a hobby, listening to music, or prayer. In addition to reducing hot flashes, making time to practice hypnotic relaxation each day is one way to express self-care.

Seek Counseling

Counseling for emotional concerns such as anxiety, depression, and stress can be very helpful, and many women with breast cancer seek counseling. Getting help starts by opening up and talking about feelings and concerns, whether they involve anxieties, depressed mood, marital relationship, sexual history, or trauma. When needed, talk with your doctor, pastor, or a clinical psychologist or mental health care provider, whoever you are most comfortable with.

❋

Women who are diagnosed with breast cancer are very likely to experience hot flashes as a result of chemotherapy, surgical removal of ovaries, or use of tamoxifen, raloxifene, or aromatase inhibitors. There is considerable evidence that the *Relief from Hot Flashes* program can significantly reduce them. In addition, it is important to recognize that a diagnosis of breast cancer can be very stressful and women are at a higher risk for anxiety and depression. If you are a breast cancer survivor, it is important to seek support and counseling as needed. Consider hypnotic relaxation as a form of self-care that can help you reduce stress as well as hot flashes.

Chapter 4

Hormone Replacement: The Risks and Benefits

In the past, hormone therapy (HT) was the standard treatment for hot flashes and was recommended to most women with moderate to severe hot flashes. It is still used by many women, but research has indicated that it can have risks as well as benefits in relieving hot flashes. It is known that hot flashes and other symptoms result from the change in hormone levels that occur during the menopause transition as ovaries produce less estrogen and progesterone. Some women can use hormone therapy (also called "menopause hormone therapy" or MHT). Estrogen is a hormone that declines during menopause and the use of estrogen relieves hot flashes and reduces vaginal dryness. However, it is now known that there can be significant health risks for some women in regard to cancer, cardiovascular disease, or stroke associated with its use. Because of this women need to make an informed decision about the use of menopause hormone therapy and carefully consider the risks as well as the benefits. In this chapter I will discuss hormone therapy: what it is, how it is used, benefits, risks, the Women's Health Initiative Study, and other considerations.

WHAT IS MENOPAUSAL HORMONE THERAPY

Hormones are substances produced by organs in the body (such as the ovaries or thyroid gland) that regulate various body functions (such as growth and menstruation). Estrogen is a particular female hormone that declines during menopause or with removal of ovaries or chemical suppression of estrogen. Menopausal hormone therapy refers to the use of medications such as estrogen and or progesterone to treat disorders caused by the estrogen deficiency.

The major forms of estrogen in these medications are derived from mares' urine (**pregnant mar**es' uri**ne**, for the brand name Premarin) or are synthetically manufactured. Many products today contain 17 beta-estradiol which is the estrogen primarily made by functioning ovaries. Hormone therapies for menopausal women are available in pill, patch, or creams. All types are absorbed into the bloodstream to prevent hot flashes and also to prevent bone loss. Hormone therapy may be prescribed to reduce hot flashes, vaginal dryness, and bone loss associated with menopause. If a woman has a uterus, then estrogen is combined with progesterone or progestin (a synthetic type of progesterone). The combination of estrogen and progesterone is used in women who have not had a hysterectomy to prevent the increased risk of uterine cancer that can occur with use of estrogen alone. If a women has had removal of the uterus, then progesterone is not indicated and estrogen alone can be utilized. Menopausal hormone therapy is not recommended to women who have a history of breast cancer, serious liver disease, thrombotic events (blood clots in their legs or lungs) or significant risk factors for heart disease or stroke.

FORMS OF MENOPAUSAL HORMONE THERAPY

To clarify, the term "menopausal hormone therapy" (MHT) is a general term that encompasses all forms of hormone treatment associated with menopause, it is sometimes also referred to as "hormone replacement therapy." There are two common types of menopausal hormone therapy.

- **Estrogen therapy (ET).** Estrogen therapy is most often prescribed for treatment of hot flashes and menopausal symptoms in women with a hysterectomy. It refers to the use of estrogen alone.
- **Estrogen plus progestin therapy (EPT).** Estrogen plus progestin (or progestogen) is a combination of these two hormones. It is most often prescribed for women who still have their uterus as described.

There are two general ways that hormone therapy can be absorbed when it is taken. Also, it can be prescribed in a number of different applications.

- Hormone therapy is available in the form of pills, patches, gel, vaginal rings, emulsion, spray, or injection. When taken in these forms it is absorbed into the bloodstream and has effects on *all parts of the body*.
- Hormone therapy can also be used in the form of a vaginal cream, ring, or tablet that is *locally applied*. In this form, estrogen is placed directly on the vaginal area or skin to treat symptoms. Locally applied vaginal estrogen can be used in very small amounts to treat only vaginal thinning and dryness. Use of these products is associated with only minimal amounts being absorbed into the bloodstream. Some vaginal products do contain higher doses of estrogen and are approved for treatment of hot flashes. The amount and type of MHT can vary depending upons the needs and preferences of a woman in consultation with her physician.

MENOPAUSAL HORMONE THERAPY RECONSIDERED

Hormone therapy has been proven effective in controlling hot flashes, rejuvenating vaginal thinning, and prevention of bone loss. Side effects such as bloating, breast soreness, headaches, and irregular vaginal bleeding can occur. By modifying the dose and cycle of the use of MHT some of these symptoms may be reduced.

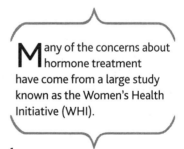

Many of the concerns about hormone treatment have come from a large study known as the Women's Health Initiative (WHI).

However, in recent years the widespread use of MHT has been reconsidered. Many of the concerns about hormone treatment have come from a large study funded by the National Institutes of Health, known as the *Women's Health Initiative (WHI)*. Therefore, it is important to be informed about the findings from this important study.

WHI STUDY

The Women's Health Initiative (WHI) was the world's largest study of postmenopausal women using hormone therapy. The study included women in the 50 to 79 age range and studied the effect of hormone therapy on older as well as younger women. It was conducted over 15 years and approximately 27,000 women were prescribed ET, EPT, or placebo pills.

This research was originally designed to examine the potential benefits of hormone therapy on aging in women, and to include a follow-up period of nine years. However, it was instead discovered that there were significant health risks, and the part of the study that involved women taking estrogen plus progesterone was abruptly stopped in July 2002, with an average follow-up period of 5.2 years.

In the WHI study, the incidence of breast cancer increased by 26% for women in the estrogen-progesterone group. In addition, the estrogen plus progesterone therapy was shown to be associated with increased cardiovascular disease and stroke. At the same time, the study showed benefits that included fewer fractures and less chance of colon cancer. However, the results indicated to the researchers that the overall risk of taking estrogen plus progesterone outweighed the benefits, and that aspect of the trial was stopped. In 2004, the estrogen only aspect of the WHI hormone trial was also stopped when it, too, showed an increased risk of stroke. However, it should be noted that the use of estrogen alone was *not* found to increase the risk of breast cancer or heart attacks. In both the estrogen plus progesterone group and the estrogen only group, risks such as cardiovascular disease and stroke were much less in women who were less than 60 years of age compared to women who were in their 60s and even 70s.

The health status of the women in the WHI study was monitored for several years after they stopped taking estrogen or estrogen plus progesterone A positive finding was that during the first three years after stopping estrogen plus progesterone, the women no longer had a greater risk of heart disease, stroke, or serious blood clots in comparison to women who never used these hormones. The women still had an increased risk of breast cancer, but the risk was lower than when they were taking estrogen in combination with progesterone. After four years, the women in the study who had stopped taking estrogen alone were found to no longer have an increased risk of stroke and the slightly lower risk of breast cancer continued.

It is noteworthy that the WHI findings are based upon only one dose and type of oral MHT (Premarin). It is not known how the WHI findings may or may not apply to smaller doses or other types of estrogen and progesterone or other delivery methods such as the patch. However, it does appear that women should generally not take MHT to protect their health, as it does not seem to prevent either heart disease or dementia. Further, because of the concerns, many women now seek more information about MHT and it is prescribed with more caution than in the past. In each woman's case it is important to consider the balance between the risks and benefits of menopausal hormone therapy.

POTENTIAL BENEFITS OF MENOPAUSAL HORMONE THERAPY

The WHI study also showed benefits from hormone therapy.

Hot Flashes

Hormone therapy reduces hot flashes by 70% to 80%. It is recognized as an effective treatment. In addition, menopausal hormone therapy generally relieves night sweats as well.

Sleep Difficulties

Sleep problems and insomnia are generally improved with menopausal hormone therapy. This may be due to the decrease in night sweats as hot flashes are less frequent.

Vaginal Dryness

Estrogen decreases vaginal dryness and pain with sexual inter-course. Hormone therapy results in improved sex drive, vaginal lubrication, and thickness of the vaginal lining. This is an important consideration for women who are sexually active.

Anxiety

The use of menopausal hormone therapy provides some benefit in regard to mood and fewer feelings of tension and anxiety

Colorectal Cancer

For women taking estrogen plus progesterone hormone therapy in the WHI study, the incidence of colorectal cancer decreased by 37%. Other factors that may contribute to the risk of colorectal cancer include genetic predisposition and use of tobacco products.

Hip Fractures

There were indications that menopausal hormone therapy may be beneficial for improving bone density, showing a small, but sig-nificant improvement. Women who were taking estrogen alone or estrogen plus progesterone were found to have a significant decrease in hip fractures.

Cholesterol Levels

It has been shown that estrogen therapy can improve cholesterol levels. However, improving cholesterol levels is not a good reason to use estrogen post-menopause because there are other medica-tions and lifestyle changes that more effectively improve choles-terol levels. Also, the pill form of estrogen can cause triglycerides to increase (an estrogen patch does not seem to have this effect, but also does not lower cholesterol as much as the pill form).

POTENTIAL RISKS OF MENOPAUSAL HORMONE THERAPY

Blood Clots

The WHI study found that taking estrogen plus progesterone increased a woman's risk of developing blood clots. This risk may be higher if the woman smokes cigarettes. Blood clots in a vein (called, deep venous thrombosis, or DVT) and blood clots in the lungs (called pulmonary emboli, or PE) increased by 41% for women taking hormone therapy. Recent studies have revealed that the estrogen patch is not associated with an increased risk of blood clots.

Breast Cancer

It is important to note that the WHI study found that the dose and oral delivery of estrogen plus progesterone increased the risk of breast cancer by up to 26%. However, it should also be noted that the use of *estrogen alone* did not increase the risk of heart attacks or breast cancer.

Cardiovascular Disease

The use of estrogen plus progesterone hormone therapy appears to increase the risk of heart disease, particularly in women who begin use more than 5 to 10 years into the menopause and have an increased risk of cardiovascular disease, including smokers, diabetics, and women with high blood pressure and high cholesterol. Healthy women initiating hormone therapy at the time they are going into the menopause are not at increased risk of heart disease. The increased risk of heart disease and stroke is particularly true for women older than age 60 and women who began use of hormones more than 10 years after becoming post-menopausal. The WHI study found that using estrogen alone did not increase the risk of heart attacks.

Endometrial Cancer

The risk for endometrial (uterine) cancer is five times higher for women who take estrogen therapy alone. On the other hand, the use of estrogen plus appropriate amounts of progesterone prevents this increased risk.

Stroke

In the WHI study, there was found to be an increase in risk for stroke for women who were taking estrogen plus progesterone and estrogen only therapy. But once again, this was primarily in women over 60 years of age and in women with health problems associated with stroke, such as high blood pressure. This is a risk that can lead to brain damage and/or physical impairments.

WEIGHING THE HEALTH RISKS AND BENEFITS

The decision whether or not to use menopausal hormone therapy is a personal one. You should consider whether or not the benefits outweigh the potential risks. The ideal candidate to consider hormone therapy is a woman with severe disruptive hot flashes who is healthy and without significant medical problems associated with heart attacks, stroke, or blood clots, and is entering the menopausal transition or within the first years after her last menstrual period. If hormone therapy is initiated, the lowest possible doses would be used to decrease side effects and potential risks. Importantly, patients who have had to have their ovaries removed before the natural age of menopause or have gone through the menopause prior to age 45 should discuss hormone therapy with their health care provider; the benefits in this young age group are much greater, as early loss of estrogen production has been associated with numerous health disorders including osteoporosis and Alzheimer's Disease.

In addition, there are considerations such as when and how long to use hormone therapy and in exactly what combination. For example, the decision about whether or not to use hormone therapy can include considerations such as:

- If and how long should I use menopausal hormone therapy?
- At what dose?
- In what form (pill, patch, gel, etc.)?
- If using menopausal hormone therapy, is it necessary to use a combination of estrogen plus progesterone or should I use estrogen alone?
- What should I do to control hot flashes *after stopping menopausal hormone therapy*?

WHO SHOULD NOT USE HORMONE THERAPY?

For some women, hormone therapy should not be used at all. There are some circumstances in which the risks clearly outweigh the benefits. This includes women who have been diagnosed with breast cancer or who have a known risk for breast cancer. The treatment for breast cancer may include surgery, chemotherapy, or radiation, or a combination of all of these. After treatment, most women are prescribed medications such as tamoxifen, raloxifene, or aromatase inhibitors. These medications stop the production of estrogen and lead to hot flashes. It is usually recommended that women who have been treated for breast cancer continue on these medications for five years. The conditions where women should not use hormone therapy include:

Women are generally urged to stop smoking as this can be a contributing factor to risks for some disease.

- Breast cancer
- Endometrial or uterine cancer
- Liver disease
- Cardiovascular disease, including a history of blood clots

Alternative, nonhormonal therapies for hot flashes should always be considered for women with any of these conditions. Additionally, behavioral changes may be encouraged; for example, smoking is a known risk factor for many diseases, and smoking cessation may be advised.

QUESTIONS TO ASK YOUR DOCTOR ABOUT MENOPAUSAL HORMONE THERAPY

If you are a woman who is experiencing menopausal symptoms, you should discuss your concerns with your physician. It is important to have regular checkups, to complete scheduled mammograms and pelvic examinations, and to monitor your medications. If you experience any unexplained uterine bleeding you should contact your physician. Some questions to ask your doctor about HT are:

- What is my risk for developing breast cancer?
- What is my risk for heart disease?
- Is menopausal hormone therapy safe for me to take and for how long?
- What is the lowest dose of HT that will improve my symptoms?
- What will help me prevent bone loss and reduce hip fractures?
- Are there lifestyle changes that I should make?
- What are the side effects?
- What alternatives to menopausal hormone therapy are available?

In discussing these questions with your physician it is helpful to know that there is no single answer for all women. Each woman should weigh her own risks and benefits. Also, there is still much that is not known about the short- and long-term use of menopausal hormone therapy. As more information becomes available, your physician may be able to provide you with guidance in making decisions that are best for you.

❊

Menopausal hormone therapy is one option for dealing with hot flashes. It is effective in reducing hot flashes and can have other benefits such as reducing the risk of colorectal cancer, hip fractures, and vaginal dryness. However, it is now known that for some women there are also potential health risks such as blood clots, breast cancer, and cardiovascular disease. Therefore, it is important for each woman to be well informed, to discuss her individual risks and needs with her physician, and to make the best decisions about her own health care. Since the results of the WHI study of hormone therapy were released, there has been great interest in identifying nonhormonal therapies such as herbs, medications, and other alternatives. In the next chapter we will review the various nonhormonal therapies and the research evidence for their effectiveness.

Chapter 5

Nonhormonal Therapies for Hot Flashes: What Do We Really Know?

A great variety of therapies and remedies have been recommended for the treatment of hot flashes. You have probably heard of, and perhaps tried, some of these, and others may be new to you. In some cases there has been quite a bit of "hype," and claims of effectiveness without much research support.

At the same time, many of these alternative therapies have been carefully evaluated in scientific studies. It is not my intent to advocate for or against any of these alternative therapies. It is my intention to present the evidence as objectively as possible.

I believe that by having as much factual information as possible you will be able to make the best decisions for yourself and avoid ineffective therapies. In a very broad way the various nonhormonal therapies fall into four categories:

1. Antidepressants
2. Other prescription drugs
3. Herbal and nonprescription remedies
4. Other alternative medicine therapies

Wherever possible, I'll present evidence for the therapies relative to placebo for comparison. I'll also share any known side effects or cautions, but in many cases the long-term effects and drug interactions are not known, so always proceed with caution and discuss any medication or remedy that you consider with your physician.

ANTIDEPRESSANTS

Antidepressant medications have been prescribed in an attempt to lower hot flashes and, in general, they have been shown to only have a modest effect over placebo (i.e., no active treatment). However, very recently the Food and Drug Administration (FDA) approved the antidepressant drug Paxil to treat hot flashes in menopausal women—after an FDA panel voted against approving the medication. The panel likely disapproved of the drug because the scientific data upon which the panel relied may not have been viewed as compelling enough for such approval.

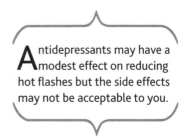

Antidepressants may have a modest effect on reducing hot flashes but the side effects may not be acceptable to you.

The current antidepressant treatments are limited in several ways. First, the antidepressants can reduce hot flashes by about 60% at best. This is about 25% to 30% less effective than hormonal treatments. Second, many women do not get this benefit. For example, in the placebo-controlled trial of venlafaxine, 37% (16 of 43) of patients did not receive a 50% or better reduction in their hot flash score. Third, it is not known how well these medications work over long periods of time, and whether side effects or sexual function changes should limit their long-term use.

Side effects of antidepressants can include such things as anxiety or nervousness, nausea, insomnia, drowsiness, diarrhea, hypertension, nightmares, dry mouth, urination problems, and loss of ability to achieve orgasm during sexual activity. Because of these side effects many women do not wish to take antidepressant medications for hot flashes over a long period of time. As with all prescriptions, your physician can discuss these concerns with you.

Effexor (Venlafaxine)

Effexor is an antidepressant drug that has been frequently prescribed for hot flashes. It is a selective norepinephrine reuptake inhibitors (SNRI) class of medication that is used in doses ranging from 37.5 mg to 150 mg per day. One of the first research investigations enrolled 28 patients, about half of whom reported a 50% reduction in hot flashes after four weeks of venlafaxine at 25 mg daily (12.5 mg twice a day). In a follow-up dose response study, 191 participants with breast cancer or risk of cancer were randomized to venlafaxine at 37.5 mg, 75 mg, or 150 mg daily for four weeks. The effect was best for those taking the 75 mg dose.

In studies of Effexor, side effects include nausea, nervousness, constipation, sleep problems, dizziness, and sexual dysfunction. In one study, nausea and vomiting led to discontinuation of the drug in about 5% to 10% of women. There is also a dose-related risk of increased high blood pressure. Contraindications include use with some other antidepressant medications.

Lexapro (Citalopram)

There is some evidence that Lexapro may provide some short-term benefit. For example, a study of Lexapro over six weeks was found to be more effective than a placebo in decreasing hot flash frequency, severity, and daily interference in a sample of 254 women. However, it may not provide much long-term benefit. One longer-term study reported null findings.

Side effects from taking Lexapro can include dry mouth, decreased energy, sexual problems, diarrhea, sweating, and, less frequently, behavioral changes.

Paxil/Brisdelle (Paroxetine)

Paxil (also marketed as Brisdelle) was recently approved by the FDA for treatment of hot flashes; however, side effects may include nausea and sleep problems. Paxil is in the selective serotonin reuptake inhibitors (SSRI) class of antidepressant medications. Paxil, in doses of 10 mg to 36.5 mg per day, improved self-reported hot flash frequency and severity in three uncontrolled trials involving cancer patients. In a randomized trial of 151 breast cancer patients, 10 mg of Paxil showed a 46% reduction in hot flash scores, and those who received 20 mg showed a 56% reduction. In another study of menopausal women there were overall decreases in hot flash scores of 62% in those taking 12.5 mg of Paxil and 65% for those taking 25 mg, compared to a 38% reduction in those who were given placebo pills.

Across studies, adverse events included nausea, decreased appetite, sleep problems, and dizziness. Contraindications include use of certain other antidepressant medications and the medication Coumadin (an anticoagulant used for prevention of blood clots). As noted earlier, the FDA has approved Paxil to treat hot flashes.

Prozac (Fluoxetine)

Prozac is another SSRI class antidepressant medication. It has been studied at the dose of 20 mg per day (this is also the dose recommended as the initial prescription to treat clinical depression). In a study of 81 women with a history of breast cancer and hot flashes, 20 mg of Prozac per day was found to be superior to placebo by about 20%. It is likely that since the magnitude of benefit was not more substantial, it has been utilized less often than other antidepressants.

Side effects have included sleep problems, dizziness, nausea, and changes in appetite. The contraindications are the same as those with Paxil and Effexor.

OTHER PRESCRIPTION DRUGS

A variety of other medications that have also been tried for treatment of hot flashes. The use of these is very limited due to side effects or lack of established effectiveness. However, they are sometimes suggested to women and information on them can be helpful.

Bellergal

Bellergal is a sedative and there is currently little support for its use in treatment of hot flashes. In one study, 66 women with hot flashes received either one tablet of Bellergal per day or a placebo. No significant group differences were seen after eight weeks of treatment. In another study, women received either Bellergal or placebo pills each day for six weeks. Hot flashes were reported to be less with the medication; however, this was not confirmed with any objective measurements.

Bellergal is potentially addictive and given the lack of solid evidence it is not generally recommended for women with hot flashes. Adverse effects can include dry mouth, visual disturbance, dizziness, and sleep disturbance among other concerns.

Clonidine

Clonidine is a medication used to treat high blood pressure, attention deficit hyperactivity disorder (ADHD), anxiety/panic disorder, and certain pain conditions. There have been several studies examining whether it could reduce hot flashes. Although clonidine appears to be more effective than placebo, concerns about its side effects have been raised. In one study, only 31% of women preferred clonidine when asked to consider its side effects. A subsequent trial in breast cancer showed that oral clonidine compared to placebo decreased hot flash frequency by only 37% at four weeks and 38% after taking the drug for eight weeks.

Concerns about clonidine are that it can lower blood pressure and heart rate. Also, adverse events have included dry mouth, dizziness, sedation, and constipation.

Gabapentin

Gabapentin is an anticonvulsant medication used to treat seizures and some chronic pain syndromes. It has also been studied for treating hot flashes. In women without cancer, four randomized controlled trials found that gabapentin in doses of 600 mg to 2,400 mg per day reduced the frequency of hot flashes by about 45%, but not much more than placebo pills. In a randomized, double-blind, placebo-controlled, multi-institutional trial of gabapentin 900 mg per day provided a 46% reduction in hot flash severity scores after eight weeks of use by breast cancer survivors. In another study, breast cancer survivors received gabapentin (900 mg per day) while either continuing or discontinuing antidepressants for hot flashes (e.g., venlafaxine, paroxetine, other). The results showed that the treatments produced similar reduction in hot flashes. Stated another way, there was not any additional benefit of adding gabapentin to antidepressant therapy.

Adverse events were not frequent, but dizziness, fatigue, eye problems, and sleep problems have been observed in some trials of gabapentin when it has been used for seizures. Hypersensitivity to the medication is a contraindication.

Megestrol Acetate

Megestrol acetate is a form of progestin. It is sometimes used to treat endometrial cancer. Though it can decrease hot flashes for some women, the safety of megestrol acetate has not yet been established, so it is not often prescribed.

Most studies indicate that herbs such as black cohosh and St. John's wort have minimal effect on hot flashes. More study is needed before they can be recommended.

HERBALS AND NONPRESCRIPTION REMEDIES

In the search for safe and effective treatments, there have been a number of herbs and food additives that have been recommended for hot flashes. You may have heard of some of these and the claims about their effectiveness. While any given individual may find some benefit, the overall research is not very supportive of their use. Most studies indicate that herbs such as black cohosh and St. John's wort have minimal effect on hot flashes. More study is needed before they can be recommended. An overview of these herbals and other nonprescription remedies follows, as you may like to try them or use them in combination with hypnotic relaxation methods.

Black Cohosh

Black cohosh is an herb derived from a North American plant. It is also known as *Cimicifuga racemosa*, and historically has been used as a remedy for menstrual problems. It has been widely studied for menopausal symptoms in women and several studies showed potential efficacy for black cohosh to reduce hot flashes. However, most of the trials showing benefit were conducted in the 1980s. Results have been mixed, but more recent randomized trials have failed to clearly demonstrate efficacy in menopausal women with hot flashes.

The most common side effects of black cohosh include headaches, vomiting, stomach complaints, and dizziness when taken in higher doses.

Dong Quai

Dong quai is an herb that is most commonly associated with Traditional Chinese Medicine (TCM). It is usually not prescribed by itself, but in combination with other herbal mixtures determined for each individual. One study has examined Dong quai for hot flashes; however, the results indicated that it is no more effective than taking a placebo.

Limited data exists on the safety of Dong quai, but it has been reported that it should not be taken in combination with the anticoagulant medication Coumadin.

Evening Primrose Oil

Evening primrose oil (*Oenothera biennis*) seeds have been used by some individuals to reduce hot flashes. To date, one randomized study examined the combination of evening primrose oil in combination with vitamin E. Women either took the combination or a placebo pill for six months. At the end of the study there was no significant improvement in hot flashes for either group.

Potential side effects of evening primrose oil can include nausea and diarrhea.

Flax Seed

Flax seed (*Linum usitatissimum*) has also been considered for treatment of hot flashes. It is believed to have an effect on estrogen and to provide antioxidant effects. However, to date there is no evidence of benefit of flax seed over placebo for hot flashes. In one study, women were randomly assigned to consume, on a daily basis, a muffin containing soy flour, ground flax seed, or wheat flour (placebo). In another study, women with hot flashes were randomized to receive two slices of bread per day containing either flax seed or wheat bran. No significant improvement in hot flashes for flax seed was seen in either of the studies.

Ginseng

Ginseng root is thought to have properties to provide energy or vitality when consumed. It is used in TCM and is popular in some cultures. One randomized study was conducted in which 384 women were assigned to take either a ginseng preparation or placebo for 14 weeks. At the end of the study it was found that ginseng had no benefit over placebo on reducing hot flashes.

Individuals who are using stimulant medications, anticoagulant medications, or certain antidepressants should avoid ginseng.

Red Clover

Red clover (*Trifolium pratense*) is a plant that is similar in chemical profile to soy. It has been employed for the treatment of menopausal symptoms. However, the results of several clinical trials have been mostly negative. One study reported a 44% reduction in hot flashes with a red clover supplement of 80 mg per day. However, a recent, well-designed study of women who used red clover at 398 mg per day did not indicate any significant benefit. At this time, red clover does not appear to be effective for hot flashes.

Adverse events from red clover have been found to be minimal; however, the long-term safety of consuming red clover has not yet been established.

Soy Isoflavones

Soy is derived from soybeans and can be consumed as a supplement or food product. Soybeans contain the isoflavones genistein and daidzein, considered by some dietitians and physicians to be useful in the prevention of cancer and endocrine disorders. Isoflavones are polyphenol compounds, produced primarily by beans and other legumes, including peanuts and chickpeas. Examples of foods high in soy isoflavones include tofu, soy milk, soy yogurt, and of course, soybeans. Soy isoflavones have been widely studied; however, well-designed clinical trials have indicated that generally hot flashes are only slightly reduced in women who consume soy products. The most common dose across studies has been between 40 mg and 80 mg per day.

The manner in which soy has an effect is not fully known. However, it is known that for some women, daidzein is converted into equol, a nonsteroidal estrogen, and while it has not been established through research, there is some concern about the safety of menopausal women consuming high doses of soy and soy-based products.

St. John's Wort

St. John's wort, also known as *Hypericum perforatum*, is a perennial herb that has been mostly studied for the treatment of depression. There has been some limited study of its use in treatment of hot flashes in women with mild to severe symptoms. The results have not been very compelling. In one study, a dose of 5,400 mg of dry herb (990 mcg hypericin, 9 mg hyperforin, 18 mg glycosides) in combination with *Vitex agnus-castus* (chaste tree/berry 500 mg of dry fruit) was not more effective than placebo in reducing hot flashes recorded on daily diaries. A recent study compared St. John's wort, 900 mg dry herb daily, to a placebo. After three months there were no significant differences in hot flash scores for St. John's wort versus placebo pills.

St. John's wort, may have interactions with medications and should be avoided in certain individuals. For example, it can result in elevated cholesterol levels and it may also affect blood glucose levels. Before using this supplement, it is important to discuss possible medication interactions with your health provider.

St. John's wort, is available in the United States and other countries; however, it is noteworthy that France has banned the use of St. John's wort due to concerns about interactions with other medications.

Vitamin E

Vitamin E has been studied as a possible treatment for hot flashes for many years. However, vitamin E therapy has not been shown to be an effective treatment. For example, in one study, 120 breast cancer patients were randomized to four weeks of vitamin E (800 IU) followed by placebo. Although there was a subjective decrease in hot flashes in the vitamin E group, the reduction was very small and only amounted to about one hot flash per day. Another study of 658 women found vitamin E (50–100 IU/d) to be no more effective than placebo.

Possible contraindications of vitamin E include patients with heart disease, diabetes, or hypertension.

OTHER ALTERNATIVE MEDICINE THERAPIES

Research into alternatives to hormone therapy and antidepressants have considered treatments such as acupuncture, magnet therapy, and reflexology. Also, exercise and yoga have been investigated as treatments for hot flashes, as well as educational and relaxation programs. Each of these therapies could be combined with hypnotic relaxation therapy depending on patient preference and interest.

Acupuncture

Acupuncture involves the placing of small needles in specific areas of the body thought to influence the flow of energy and health. The evidence for acupuncture in relieving hot flashes is mixed. Most of the studies have been remarkable for an overall lack of supporting evidence for the use of acupuncture for hot flashes. One recently published study indicated that women receiving individualized acupuncture had significant improvement in hot flashes compared to no-treatment after 12 weeks. However, these benefits were not sustained 6 or 12 months later. Another study compared acupuncture to Effexor (venlafaxine) in treating hot flashes in 50 breast cancer survivors. That study found acupuncture to be comparable to the medication in reducing the frequency and severity of hot flashes. Therefore, it appears that acupuncture may offer some relief to patients; however, the long-term benefit may be lacking unless the acupuncture treatments continue.

> Acupuncture may offer some relief; however, the long-term benefit may be lacking unless the acupuncture treatments continue.

Biofeedback and Relaxation Training

Biofeedback therapy is a method in which a device is used to measure physical responses such as muscle tension, body temperature, heart rate, blood pressure, or even brain waves. These responses are provided as "feedback" to the patient along with instruction in the use of relaxation exercises. It has been shown that biofeedback and relaxation can be useful in treatment of tension and migraine headaches, pain problems, anxiety, insomnia, and a host of psychophysiological disorders. Also, relaxation training has been found to be of benefit for treating hot flashes. For example, in one small study four women were able to reduce self-reported hot flashes from 41% to 90% through the use of temperature biofeedback, when provided with instruction in relaxation and mental imagery that included thoughts of coolness.

Other interventions that have been studied have included progressive muscle relaxation, relaxation combined with temperature control biofeedback training, and at-home relaxation audiotapes. These methods have all been shown to be of significant benefit in achieving reductions in hot flash frequency and severity. Also, it is noteworthy that hypnotic relaxation therapy includes a component of relaxation and uses mental imagery for coolness as well as other components described in detail in later chapters.

Relaxation-based interventions may be of benefit to many patients. The research on hypnotic relaxation therapy has been most persuasive, with findings of 68% to 80% reduction in hot flashes. Relaxation-based therapies can be integrated with most other treatments.

Exercise

The health benefits of exercise are well known. Exercise can improve quality of life, energy, and cardiovascular health, can reduce risk of cancer, and plays an important role in weight loss. However, there is mixed evidence about whether or not exercise significantly improves hot flashes. There have been only a few studies of exercise for treatment of hot flashes and most of these have found

> Hypnotic relaxation therapy has been most persuasive, with findings of 68% to 80% reduction in hot flashes.

no differences between weekly exercise and no treatment.

In fact, one study found that after 12 months with exercise there was a significant increase in hot flash severity. It is possible that exercise may increase core body temperature and trigger hot flashes. However, the relationship between hot flashes and exercise may be more complex, as another study found that it could decrease hot flashes for some women. A recent study suggests that whether exercise increases or decreases hot flashes may depend on a woman's preexisting fitness level.

A recent study of 92 healthy women found that immediately after moderate-intensity aerobic exercise, they reported significantly fewer hot flashes. However, this study also revealed that women who were not as physically fit reported more hot flashes when they participated in aerobic exercise, indicating that fitness levels should be considered when recommending exercise to deal with hot flashes.

Magnet Therapy

Magnets can be worn and placed on specific areas of the body. Some people have a strong belief in the benefit of magnet therapy, and magnets have been used for many years as an alternative medical treatment. However, there is little to no evidence to support the use of magnets to reduce hot flashes. One randomized study investigated the use of magnets to treat hot flashes in 15 postmenopausal breast cancer survivors. The study did not find any significant relief from hot flashes for patients using magnets.

Mindfulness-Based Stress Reduction

Mindfulness refers to a meditative practice that emphasizes awareness of the present moment. In recent years a program called mindfulness-based stress reduction (MBSR) has become very popular and the subject of several clinical research studies. MBSR includes the practice of mindfulness meditation and yoga as well as educational components.

MBSR usually involves eight weekly classes lasting two and one-half hours each, an all-day weekend retreat, and at-home practice. Participants are taught principles of acceptance and to observe themselves in a nonjudgmental manner as a part of the practice. MBSR has been shown to have beneficial effects on reducing stress, chronic pain, and dependence on addictive substances, as well as in developing coping skills.

Two studies have been conducted on the use of MBSR for hot flashes. In a pilot study, 15 women attended an eight-week MBSR program for the treatment of hot flashes. The results showed a 40% reduction in hot flash severity, and feelings of improvement were reported as to quality of life. Following this initial study, a large randomized controlled trial was conducted. One hundred and ten women with moderate to severe hot flashes completed a standard eight-week MBSR intervention. The participants who received MBSR reported benefits in regard to quality of life and coping with stress; however, there was not a reduction in hot flashes and only a 15% reduction in "hot flashes bother" (the degree to which the women were bothered or distressed by their hot flashes). After three months of MBSR practice 25 minutes per day, the women reported a slight improvement, with a 27% reduction in hot flash bother. Although, MBSR has potential health benefits in regard to stress management, it cannot be recommended as an effective treatment for hot flashes.

Paced Respiration

Paced respiration is a relaxation exercise in which individuals are instructed in slow breathing using a particular technique. During the practice of paced respiration one takes six to eight slow, deep breaths per minute while inhaling through the nose and slowly exhaling through the mouth. It is easy to learn and practice and is similar in some ways to breathing techniques taught in Lamaze classes.

In one small study paced respiration was effective in reducing physiologically recorded and/or self-reported hot flashes. In that study, the instruction in paced breathing was delivered during one-on-one, biweekly, hour-long laboratory sessions, and the women in the study practiced twice daily. However, a recent large-scale randomized controlled trial of paced respiration failed to find any significant benefit. These recent findings suggest paced respiration is unlikely to be an effective treatment for hot flashes among women during menopause or for breast cancer survivors.

Psychoeducation and Cognitive-Behavioral Programs

Psychoeducational interventions involve a variety of components such as teaching women about the physiology of hot flashes, how to identify specific thoughts that may lead to anxiety, and ways of coping with stress and symptoms. Psychoeductional and cognitive–behavioral programs have been used to help people cope with stress, manage depression, and reduce chronic pain. Psychoeducation is a component of many programs. However, there is not much evidence that psychoeducation alone is an effective treatment for hot flashes.

In one study, 96 women with a history of breast cancer were randomized to receive either a cognitive–behavioral intervention or just continue with their usual medical care. The treatment involved education about hot flashes, paced respiration, and cognitive and behavioral strategies to help the women cope with stress. After attending classes for nine weeks the women reported a reduction in hot flashes. The intervention was time- and resource-intensive to deliver; however, it was generally well-received.

Reflexology

Reflexology is a type of massage of the feet or hands. Practitioners of reflexology claim that areas of the feet and hands correspond to certain organs, glands, and parts of the body. It is believed that applying massage and pressure to the hands and feet can promote relaxation, healing, and treatment of specific symptoms or disorders. While reflexology is generally experienced as pleasant, it is unlikely to improve hot flashes. One randomized trial of reflexology for hot flashes has been conducted. In this study, 76 women with hot flashes were randomized to receive either foot reflexology or a routine foot massage for six weekly sessions. Each session lasted for about 45 minutes. There was no difference in the two treatments for improving the frequency or severity of hot flashes, nor was there any difference in anxiety or depression. At this time, reflexology has not been shown to be of significant benefit in treatment of hot flashes.

Yoga

Yoga is an ancient Eastern tradition dating back over 5000 years. It is practiced by millions of people and involves a combination of body postures, exercise, focus on breathing, and meditation. Yoga may reduce stress and anxiety, depression, hypertension, and chronic pain. More generally, the practice of yoga can increase strength, flexibility, and overall fitness, and promote relaxation.

There are many different styles of yoga; however the two most popular styles practiced in the United States are *Hatha yoga* and *Inyengar yoga*. Goals of Hatha yoga include bringing about relaxation, developing inner meditation techniques, achieving harmony of the mind and body, increasing strength, and opening channels for the flow of consciousness, which are referred to as *nadis*.

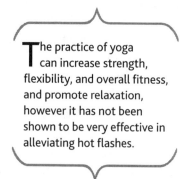

The practice of yoga can increase strength, flexibility, and overall fitness, and promote relaxation, however it has not been shown to be very effective in alleviating hot flashes.

Iyengar yoga was developed by Yogacharya Iyengar, who founded his yoga institute in 1975. It emphasizes correct body alignment, and practitioners may use various props such as wooden blocks and chairs to assist them in achieving correct movements or postures. Also, Iyengar yoga emphasizes the practice of meditation. The meditative state of Iyengar yoga has been described as a trance-like state of relaxation.

While yoga has a number of benefits, it has not been shown to be very effective in alleviating hot flashes. For example, in one study 37 women with hot flashes were randomly assigned to either eight weeks of yoga or a wait-list control. The reduction in hot flashes was not significant. There was a reduction of 31%, but this was similar to the placebo response found in other studies.

❋

There is a wide range of nonhormonal therapies available to treat hot flashes; however, most of these therapies have not been shown to be very effective in reducing them. Some of these therapies, such as medications and some herbs or supplements, may have some significant side effects and should be used only with caution. Other alternative therapies such as yoga, exercise, and acupuncture may be of general health benefit and would probably do you no harm. Hypnotic relaxation therapy is the most successful option for reducing hot flashes and it can be used in conjunction with all traditional and alternative approaches. Knowing the facts will help you craft the most effective and personalized approach for dealing with your hot flashes.

In the next chapter we will begin to discuss hypnotic relaxation therapy in more detail so you can begin to use it to reduce your hot flashes.

Chapter 6

Hypnotic Relaxation Therapy: What It Is and Why You Need It

Hypnotic relaxation therapy has been shown to be very effective in helping women to reduce hot flashes without using hormones or drugs. It is a safe and effective method that has been used by many women in my practice. It is also a new and innovative method for reducing hot flashes, and many people are unaware of hypnotic relaxation therapy and how it works. Think of hypnotic relaxation as a tool. In and of itself, a tool cannot change anything. If you look at a wrench or hammer, they have no effect without being put to use. However, when we learn to use a tool, it can be very effective.

Most people have heard of "hypnosis" or some other relaxation methods, such as meditation. However, the term hypnosis has been around for a long time and its representation in numerous movies and television shows has been filled with misconceptions and misinformation. In this chapter, I will address the misconceptions, give you information on the development of hypnotic relaxation therapy, and describe the relevant research. It is important for you to know exactly what hypnotic relaxation therapy is and how it can work for you.

DEFINITION

Hypnotic relaxation therapy is a mind–body therapy involving therapeutic relaxation, mental imagery, and positive suggestions. What do I mean by mind–body? In everyday waking consciousness there is a connection between the mind and the body. We are not always aware of this connection, but it occurs in both positive and negative ways. For example, if you are worried about something those worries can be translated into physical tension, such as tight muscles, achy, tense shoulders, or tension headaches. Most people have experienced this connection between the mind and the body. Through hypnotic relaxation therapy, you can experience the mind–body connection in a positive way by using your mind to calm and relax your body.

During a session of hypnotic relaxation therapy, you become very deeply relaxed and enter a hypnotic state. This state is similar to what it feels like when you are drifting off to sleep. While in this state, you are able to vividly imagine and are given therapeutic suggestions to relieve your hot flashes, for example, of being in a very cool place.

The hypnotic state is in a sense an "altered state of consciousness" which means that you are very absorbed in the imagined or suggested experiences. For example, if I suggest that you imagine being in a flower garden, you can see, feel, and experience being in the garden. An everyday example of the hypnotic state is when we go to the movies or watch a television program. If the movie is very interesting and engaging, we can "suspend critical judgment" and just enjoy the movie. At such times, we can feel emotions, react to the movie imagery, and time can seem to pass very quickly. That is what the hypnotic state feels like. It is not mind control.

The term "hypnotic relaxation therapy" is used to signify the scientific use of hypnotic methods to achieve the hypnotic state, and it identifies the specific program provided in this book. It is also the term preferred by some patients because it easily distinguishes it from the myths and misconceptions associated with the term "hypnosis."

> A goal of hypnotic relaxation therapy is to help you learn to relax and use mental imagery to reduce hot flashes.

HISTORY

Methods of hypnotic relaxation and mental imagery have been used since ancient times. The history of hypnosis is usually traced to Franz Anton Mesmer who was a physician during the 18th century. Mesmer published a doctoral dissertation in 1766 titled, *On the Influence of the Planets on the Human Body,* which discusses the impact the moon and planets were believed to have on the human body. This came about as a result of his theory of "animal magnetism."

In 1774, while treating a patient, Mesmer had her drink a mixture containing iron and attached magnets to parts of her body. He believed that in doing so he could produce what he described as an "artificial tide" as the patient described feeling relaxed. The patient also reported that her symptoms were relieved for several hours. Mesmer eventually came to understand that the magnets were not necessary to achieve the reported results; however, he mistakenly thought that *he* had contributed to the animal magnetism by passing his hands in front of the patient. He soon stopped using the magnets in his practice and promoted the use of what he called animal magnetism.

In his practice, Mesmer would sit facing his patient with their knees nearly touching. He would look intently into the patient's eyes and move his hands from the patient's shoulder down the arms. He would then press his fingers in the area just below the patient's diaphragm, and many patients reported "peculiar sensations" or experienced convulsions that were interpreted as "crisis"—the element which was supposed to bring about the cure. He would conclude his session by having an assistant play music on a glass armonica, an instrument made of glass bowls graduated in size.

During his time, Mesmer became very popular and had a thriving practice in Paris, but his theory was often challenged. Following the French Revolution, Mesmer went to Switzerland and continued to practice animal magnetism until his death in 1815.

Benjamin Franklin and other prominent figures of the time conducted an investigation on Mesmer and his patients. It was concluded that the effect of Mesmerism was due to suggestion and the use of imagination. The idea of animal magnetism was disproven.

However, even today we use the term "mesmerized" to describe being fascinated. Many of the myths about hypnosis can be traced back to Mesmer.

During the early 19th century, James Braid, a physician in Scotland, began using some similar methods of relaxation and mental imagery to help his patients. He observed that during such sessions his patients appeared relaxed with eyes closed. He thought they were in a kind of sleep and he coined the word "hypnosis" from the Greek word *hypnos,* meaning sleep. He later realized that the patients were not actually asleep.

Methods of hypnosis then became more popular and were used in neurology and even in surgery. There were several cases reported in which patients were able to enter a very deep hypnotic state and undergo surgical procedures using these methods. We now know that people who are highly hypnotizable are in fact able to manage pain and can accomplish a great deal of control when provided with proper guidance.

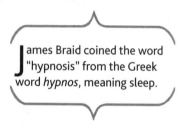

James Braid coined the word "hypnosis" from the Greek word *hypnos*, meaning sleep.

A turning point in the history of hypnosis came when Sigmund Freud studied hypnosis and worked with the famous neurologist Jean Marie Charcot. Freud used hypnosis with many of his patients before he developed the methods of psychoanalysis. He essentially rejected hypnosis in favor of his increasing interest in psychoanalysis. With this, hypnosis again lapsed into disfavor and was taken up by performers as entertainment. This is the period when many of the myths and misconceptions about hypnosis emerged and filtered into popular culture. Even today, it is possible to see "hypnosis shows" in Las Vegas and at county fairs.

Beginning in the 1930s and 1940s there was an increased interest in the study of hypnosis, and following World War II, hypnosis became the subject of serious scientific research. In 1949, the Society of Clinical and Experimental Hypnosis was established and brought together top scientists and physicians for serious investigation. Additional professional societies followed, including the American Society of Clinical Hypnosis in 1959 and the Society for Psychological Hypnosis, a division of the American Psychological Association, in 1969.

Research has now been conducted in the use of hypnotherapy for the treatment of pain, anxiety, insomnia, irritable bowel syndrome, and a host of other problems. In 1996, the National Center for Complementary and Alternative Medicine (NCCAM) of the National Institutes of Health (NIH) endorsed hypnotherapy in the treatment of chronic pain, anxiety, and insomnia. The support of NCCAM has further motivated research through funding well-designed clinical trials of mind–body medicine including hypnosis. This has significantly influenced the movement toward increased use of sound science in evaluation of hypnotherapy's effects and has shifted hypnosis research toward greater rigor through use of randomized clinical trials. Leading researchers include David Patterson and Mark Jensen at the University of Washington; Guy Montgomery at Mount Sinai School of Medicine in New York; David Spiegel at Stanford University; Olafur Palsson and William Whitehead at the University of North Carolina School of Medicine; Steven Lynn at Binghamton University, State University of New York; Arreed Barabasz at Washington State University; and Elvira Lang at Harvard University. My own research, which I describe in the following sections, was funded in part by the NIH, from both the NCCAM and from the National Cancer Institute.

FOUNDATIONS OF HYPNOTIC RELAXATION THERAPY

The foundation of hypnotic relaxation therapy is science. It is based upon research that has shown that people can benefit from therapeutic relaxation. When people enter a state of deep relaxation there are a number of positive changes that occur in the body. There is a decrease in muscle tension and a slowing of the heart rate, hormonal effects associated with the "stress response" begin to decrease, and there are sometimes changes in the immune system. The body begins to function in a calm and balanced manner, and a person begins to feel rested. Studies have shown that when individuals are given a suggestion to imagine certain objects, the areas of the brain associated with "seeing" the object become activated.

In a hypnotic state, we are able to process experiences at both conscious and unconscious levels of awareness. The conscious level of awareness refers to our ability to think in a critical and analytical way. For example, when we fill out our tax forms we are using the conscious mind. In that instance we need to think in a critical manner. However, we also have the ability to respond with our feelings. The unconscious mind tends to respond to emotions. It is influenced by "vibes" and feelings, images, stories, and metaphors. During a hypnotic relaxation induction we become more deeply relaxed and we have more awareness of the unconscious mind.

As you begin to use hypnotic relaxation you will learn to "let go" of the critical thinking and respond to the suggestions and mental imagery. As you do, you will find that the responses to suggestions for relaxation and control will feel more and more effortless. They will seem automatic and easy.

RESEARCH ON HYPNOTIC RELAXATION THERAPY FOR HOT FLASHES

There have been a number of research trials in which the hypnotic relaxation therapy program for hot flashes has been studied. This research includes case studies, retrospective clinical studies, and randomized trials with both breast cancer survivors and postmenopausal women. In each study the findings have been that the program reduces hot flashes by 70% to 80% *on average.*

A large-scale clinical study was conducted to determine if hypnotic relaxation therapy could reduce hot flashes in postmenopausal women with *moderate to very severe* hot flashes. I also wanted to see if the intervention would improve both self-reported hot flashes and those that could be measured through physiological monitoring. To do this I undertook a five-year study and enrolled 187 postmenopausal women into a large randomized clinical trial. The study was funded by the NCCAM of the NIH. In order for women to be in the study they had to be having 50 or more hot flashes per week or a minimum of seven hot flashes per day. In addition, they had to stop all other treatments for hot flashes, including hormone therapy, antidepressants, herbs, and so on. They also had to agree to keep daily diaries to record their hot flashes and to wear special monitors (called Biolog recorders) that record the physiological events and changes that go along with a hot flash.

Approximately half of the women received the hypnotic relaxation therapy program and the other half received "structured attention." The structured attention involved meeting individually with a research therapist for five visits, each lasting about 45 to 60 minutes. At each visit the women discussed their hot flashes and received supportive counseling, but did not receive any hypnotic relaxation therapy.

The women who completed the hypnotic relaxation therapy program reported significantly reduced hot flashes. After five weeks the hot flashes had decreased by about 70%, and the decrease continued, reaching 80% after three months in the program.

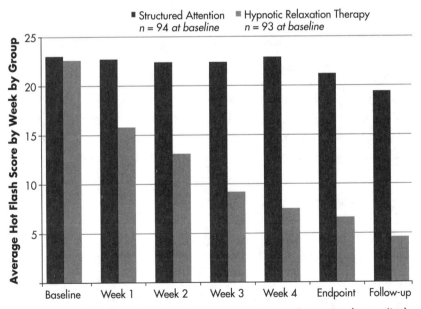

Comparison of hypnotic relaxation therapy versus structured attention (counseling) to reduce hot flashes among postmenopausal women

In addition to reducing hot flashes, the women who completed the hypnotic relaxation therapy program experienced other benefits as well. They reported fewer feelings of anxiety and stress. Their sleep quality was improved. They reported significant decreases in the degree to which hot flashes interfered with daily activities for all measures including work, social activities, leisure activities, sleep, mood, concentration, relations with others, sexuality, enjoyment of life, and overall quality of life.

For example, one of the participants, Kelley, had been on estrogen replacement therapy for 15 years before she began the program. She was having 10 to 12 hot flashes each day between the moderate and the moderately severe range. According to Kelley, "At night I could not sleep and it didn't matter if it was winter, summer, spring, or fall, I had to have on an oscillating fan and the ceiling fan. I would go to sleep, then I would throw the covers off. Then I would turn over and I would pull them back because I would get cold. During the day, at work, all of a sudden, I would feel drenched. I'd want to pull my skin off. Hypnotic relaxation therapy has completely made my life wonderful. It's very relaxing. I look forward to the sessions. By the second or third week in the study, I experienced a reduction in my hot flashes. I have been hot flash free for months now."

In this book you will receive the same materials, diaries, and audio recordings that were available to the women in the study. These materials will provide you with the tools to use so that you will see the same success as the women in the research study.

NEXT STEPS

You now have an understanding of hypnotic relaxation therapy and how it can reduce hot flashes. The next step is to learn how to measure hot flashes, stress, and sleep, and to track your progress once you begin the program. In the following chapters, in the section titled "First Things First," you will learn how to complete a Hot Flash Daily Diary, rate your sleep, and assess the effect of hot flashes on your mood, relationships, and quality of life. It is important to fill out all of the questionnaires and learn how to keep a Hot Flash Daily Diary *before* starting the use of hypnotic relaxation therapy and the audio recordings provided with this book.

Follow all of the steps and you will achieve the very best results!

FIRST THINGS FIRST

Chapter 7

Measuring Your Hot Flashes

As with any program that you use to improve your health, it is important to be able to *see* the improvement; and keeping a record of your experience is a good way to do so. The first step in this program is to identify how often you experience hot flashes and how severe they are. You will be able to do this by keeping a Hot Flash Daily Diary for seven days prior to begin-

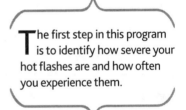

The first step in this program is to identify how severe your hot flashes are and how often you experience them.

ning your practices with the recordings. This will help you to determine your beginning, or *baseline*, hot flash information.

KEEPING A HOT FLASH DAILY DIARY

To measure your hot flashes, you will use a Hot Flash Daily Diary, which will include the following information:

- Days of the week and dates
- Total number, or *frequency*, of hot flashes
- The *severity* or intensity of each hot flash (mild, moderate, severe, or very severe)
- Calculation of your weekly *hot flash score*.

With this information, you will be able to keep track of the percentage of reduction in your hot flashes each week.

Here is a blank Hot Flash Daily Diary:

Baseline
HOT FLASH DAILY DIARY

| Date | Make a mark for each hot flash to indicate mild, moderate, severe, or very severe | | | | Total # of Hot Flashes Today | NOTES (Use this space to record possible triggers or other information relating to trends you may notice about your hot flashes) |
	MILD	MODE-RATE	SEVERE	VERY SEVERE		
MON / /	___	___	___	___		
TUES / /	___	___	___	___		
WEDS / /	___	___	___	___		
THURS / /	___	___	___	___		
FRI / /	___	___	___	___		
SAT / /	___	___	___	___		
SUN / /	___	___	___	___		
TOTALS						

Severity Descriptors

Mild	Lasts <5 minutes; uncomfortable warmth; mild discomfort; no need for action
Moderate	Up to 15 minutes; warm, clammy skin; increased heart rate; some sweating; agitated; embarrassed; use fan, remove clothes, etc.
Severe	Up to 20 minutes; very hot; increased heart rate; unusual sensation over skin; sweating; anxiety; embarrassment; activity interruption
Very severe	Up to 45 minutes; extreme heat; rolling perspiration; increased heart rate; nausea; extreme distress; difficulty functioning; need to take cold shower or hold ice on skin

Days of the Week and Dates

Use the Hot Flash Daily Diary to record the date and day of the week. It is very important that you begin each day at the same time so that you have seven equal days of measure. This helps to ensure an accurate number of daily hot flashes. If you begin your diary on Wednesday at 8:00 a.m., you will enter the date beside "Wed" and that row will include all of the hot flashes you experience until Thursday morning at 8:00 a.m.

Frequency of Hot Flashes

The number of hot flashes that you experience can vary from day to day; therefore, recording the *frequency* of your hot flashes is an important measure, especially as you attempt to identify *triggers* (something that initiates or precedes a hot flash; more on this in chapter 8). To measure the frequency of your hot flashes, you will keep a running count of every hot flash you have. This is done each day. You may want to begin your "day" at your usual waking time, or you can start a new day at noon, or when you go to bed. The *begin time* is not as important as

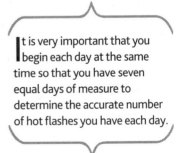

It is very important that you begin each day at the same time so that you have seven equal days of measure to determine the accurate number of hot flashes you have each day.

it is to consistently begin each new day at the *exact same time*. At the end of each week you will add up the total number of hot flashes for each day and the total for the week. You can reference the blank Hot Flash Daily Diary to see where these totals are recorded.

Total Number of Hot Flashes for Each Day: The column titled "Total # of Hot Flashes Today" will be calculated at the end of each day by totaling all of the columns indicating severity.

Total Number of Hot Flashes for the Week: After seven days, you will be able fill in the "Total" row at the bottom of the diary. The final row is the sum of all of your hot flashes for the seven-day period. The first four columns divide your hot flashes into the four categories of severity. The final column is the overall total. This "Total" can be calculated by adding the one column of daily totals and/or the row of severity totals.

Severity of Hot Flashes

As you've probably been suffering with them for a while, you know by now that your hot flashes come in various shapes and sizes. They range in description from "a hot raging feeling from deep within my body that pushes its way out," to "a crawling heat on my scalp," to "a warm sensation." A hot flash can last from a few seconds to several minutes; it can be mildly uncomfortable or it can make you want to dive into an icy bath.

Because of this, it is important to measure the *severity* of a hot flash in definable terms with clear criteria for what is considered a "mild," "moderate," "severe," or "very severe" hot flash. These terms are defined using four criteria: duration, physical symptoms, emotional symptoms, and action needed (see table on following page). This information is very important as you establish your baseline hot flash information and track it to see your progress as you go through the treatment program.

Using the defining terms to identify hot flash severity, you will decide each time you have a hot flash how it should be recorded: mild, moderate, severe, or very severe. This measure is important, as it provides a visual that indicates change in how long the hot flash lasts, how it affects you, both physically and emotionally, and how you are able to manage the hot flash as it occurs. As you begin, use the table to determine the severity of each hot flash. Place a mark for the hot flash in the appropriate "severity" column, grouping them in sets of five—it makes it easier to count, especially if you are experiencing many hot flashes each day.

Definitions of Hot Flash Severity

	GENERAL DESCRIPTION	DURATION	PHYSICAL SYMPTOMS	EMOTIONAL SYMPTOMS	ACTION NEEDED
MILD	Sensation of heat without sweating	Less than 5 min	Warmth; uncomfortable feeling; red face	Mild discomfort	Usually, no action taken
MODERATE	Sensation of heat with sweating that does not cause you to stop your current activity	Up to 15 min	Head, neck, ears, or whole body felt warm; tense, tight muscles, clammy (wet) skin; a change in heart rate or rhythm (heart speeds up or changes beat); some sweating; dry mouth	Agitation, drained of energy, embarrassed in front of others, tired, annoyed	Used a fan, awakened at night, uncovered, removed clothing, drank water, opened the window
SEVERE (Note: All night sweats should be recorded on the Hot Flash Daily Diary as "severe")	Sensation of intense heat with extreme sweating that causes you to stop your current activity	Up to 20 min	Warmth, may be described as a raging furnace, change in heart rate or rhythm, faintness, headache, severe sweating, unusual sensation over skin, chest heaviness	Embarrassment, anxiety, feelings of having a panic attack	Stopped what was being done at the time, awakened at night and removed covers, removed clothes, opened windows, kept the house cooler, used fans
VERY SEVERE	Sensation of very extreme heat (boiling eruption) rolling perspiration and behavioral disturbance	Up to 45 min	Boiling heat, rolling sweat, difficulty breathing, faintness, dizziness, cramping, change in heart rate or rhythm, nausea	Distressed feelings, have the urge to escape, have difficulty functioning	Awakened frequently at night, changed sheets and pajamas, took a cold shower, held ice on skin

Total Number in Each Severity Level: At the bottom of the Hot Flash Daily Diary, you will see a row marked "Total." For this row, you will calculate, at the end of the week, the number of hot flashes within each severity column. This is a measure you will likely see shift from being more heavily weighted on the right (severe, very severe) to the left (mild, moderate) as you go through this program.

Notes

You may want to make some notes regarding your hot flashes. For example, on some days you may observe a trend about your hot flashes on certain days. These may be activities, emotions, or situations that could affect your hot flashes. To identify this information, your Hot Flash Daily Diary includes a "Notes" column for you to record any information you notice about when your hot flashes occur (i.e., what you were doing, eating, or drinking, or how you were feeling when you experienced the hot flash). As you begin, you may not detect any special association between your hot flashes and your activities, or you may realize some very clear relationships.

Now I will show you how to calculate your weekly hot flash scores.

HOW TO CALCULATE YOUR HOT FLASH SCORE

At the end of each week you will be asked to calculate an overall "hot flash score" for the week. The hot flash score represents a combination of the frequency and severity of hot flashes for the week. To determine your hot flash score you will need to refer to your Hot Flash Daily Diary, where each severity category is given a point value.

- one point for a mild hot flash
- two points for a moderate hot flash
- three points for a severe hot flash
- four points for a very severe hot flash

Once you determine the values of each severity, simply add them to determine your hot flash score.

Example:

Mild:	10 hot flashes × 1 = 10
Moderate:	11 hot flashes × 2 = 22
Severe:	10 hot flashes × 3 = 30
Very severe:	3 hot flashes × 4 = 12

74 = Weekly Hot Flash Score

EMILY

Emily was a 57-year-old woman who was experiencing moderate to severe hot flashes. She was referred to me by her family physician for treatment of her hot flashes. Emily reported that she found concentration difficult, she rarely had a "good night's sleep," her mood shifted frequently, and the physical aspects of hot flashes (sweating, flushing, etc.) were an embarrassment in her work as a teacher. She felt that the hot flashes were the reason for some of the other problems she was experiencing, and it had become so severe that her daily life was affected in such a way that there were times that she could barely function.

Over the next several chapters I will share with you Emily's progress on the *Relief from Hot Flashes* program, starting from baseline to the end of the program. I will show you Emily's hot flash daily diaries and other information on a week-to-week basis as examples. I will also share more about Emily, some problems she encountered, her successes, and her overall experience as she completed her five weeks of hypnotic relaxation therapy. You will be able to compare your progress to Emily's.

In the beginning, Emily was asked to complete her baseline Hot Flash Daily Diary. For one week prior to our first therapy session, Emily recorded her hot flashes to determine how many hot flashes she was experiencing each day and how severe they were. As you can see, the majority of her hot flashes fell more to the right of her diary in the "Severe" and "Very Severe" columns. Additionally, from her notes, you can recognize that stress appears to be a predominant trigger for Emily's hot flashes. Her sleep is also affected, as she records multiple night sweats each night.

Emily's Baseline
HOT FLASH DAILY DIARY

| Date | Make a mark for each hot flash to indicate mild, moderate, severe, or very severe | | | | Total # of Hot Flashes Today | NOTES (Use this space to record possible triggers or other information relating to trends you may notice about your hot flashes) |
	MILD	MODE-RATE	SEVERE	VERY SEVERE		
MON 7/23/xx	I	II	II	I	6	Stress; getting girls ready for softball game Woke 2 X's with night sweats
TUES 7/24/xx	II	II	IIII		9	Stress; shopping Putting on my makeup Woke 3 X's with sweats
WEDS 7/25/xx	II	I	III	I	7	Stress; looking for keys Putting on makeup Woke 3X's with night sweats
THURS 7/26/xx	II	III	IIII	I	10	Stress; working on the budget, ball game, other stuff; makeup Woke 4X's with night sweats
FRI 7/27/xx	II	II	IIII	I	9	Stress: shopping, grandkids Alcohol: wine Woke 3X's with sweats
SAT 7/28/xx	I	III	III	I	8	Stress: shopping with grandkids, cleaning house for party. Woke 3X's with sweats
SUN 7/29/xx	III	IIII	IIII	I	12	Stress; party preparations, then party: Alcohol-wine Woke 4X's with night sweats
TOTALS	13	17	25	6	61	

Severity Descriptors

Mild	Lasts <5 minutes; uncomfortable warmth; mild discomfort; no need for action
Moderate	Up to 15 minutes; warm, clammy skin; increased heart rate; some sweating; agitated; embarrassed; use fan, remove clothes, etc.
Severe	Up to 20 minutes; very hot; increased heart rate; unusual sensation over skin; sweating; anxiety; embarrassment; activity interruption
Very severe	Up to 45 minutes; extreme heat; rolling perspiration; increased heart rate; nausea; extreme distress; difficulty functioning; need to take cold shower or hold ice on skin

Though she knew the hot flashes were bad, Emily was quite surprised that she was having as many as she was. In her words:

"I think I just tried to ignore them and I've been having them so long, I guess to some degree I was. They are just such a part of my life that I go through the motions without really realizing how many times a day I'm having hot flashes."

You may also be surprised at how frequent and how severe your hot flashes are, but this awareness will help you to identify key information to use as a measure to record improvement.

Emily's Baseline Hot Flash Score

An example of how to calculate your Hot Flash Score is given here, using the entries on Emily's baseline Hot Flash Diary.

Mild:	13 hot flashes	× 1 = 13
Moderate:	17 hot flashes	× 2 = 34
Severe:	25 hot flashes	× 3 = 75
Very severe:	6 hot flashes	× 4 = 24

146 = Emily's baseline Hot Flash Score

RECORDING YOUR HOT FLASHES

Getting started is easy. With your baseline Hot Flash Daily Diary in hand, you will begin by filling in the dates for the first week.

Note the time you are beginning your first "day," and simply begin marking hot flashes. At night, place your diary beside your bed or at the breakfast table, so you will remember to record your nightly hot flashes as soon as you wake up each morning. In the beginning you may spend a little time determining the best way

You may be surprised at how frequent and how severe your hot flashes are, but this awareness will help you to identify key information that you will use as a measure to record improvement.

for you to keep up with and mark your Hot Flash Daily Diary, but be patient with yourself and with the program. You will find that this baseline step proves to be very important as you move forward through the program. This step not only gives you a point of reference to use as you begin to see improvement, but it also gives you the opportunity to familiarize yourself with the hot flashes and how they impact your overall life.

COUNTING THEM ALL!

The task of carrying a Hot Flash Daily Diary with you 24/7 for several weeks may seem a bit daunting. But it's really not as difficult as it may sound to accurately and completely keep up with your hot flashes. My patients have used the following techniques. You could try one of these or come up with your own method.

> *Janice:* "I work as a pharmacy tech and it is VERY fast-paced all day long. There is no way I can take time to pull out a diary and mark it every time I have a hot flash! Some days, I may have 9 or 10. The way I keep up with them is that I begin my morning with a piece of white tape on my arm with mild, mod, sev, and very sev written on it. Then as I go through my day, I can simply make a mark on the tape every time I have a hot flash, because I ALWAYS have a pen with me. Then when I get home, I just transfer all of the hot flashes over to my diary."

> *Beverly:* "I don't have a problem keeping up with my hot flashes during the day because I'm home all day, and besides, I don't really have that many during the day. The nights are a different story though! It seems like I don't sleep at all, because I'm continuously tossing and turning, throwing off covers, pulling up covers, and even having to get up sometimes to stand in front of the air conditioner. By the time my alarm goes off, I couldn't tell you how many I've had, but I know I've had a LOT! So what I do is…I keep a little dish of pennies on the table by my bed. Then every time I wake up

during the night with a hot flash, I just take one of the pennies from the dish and place it on the table. Next morning, I just count the pennies and record them on my diary under severe, since all of the nighttime flashes are definitely severe."

Another one of my patients, Sandra, used a variation of Beverley's method. She used premoistened towelettes to wipe her face each time she had a hot flash at night. In the morning, she counted her used towelettes.

You can be flexible in the method you use to count and record your hot flashes, and you should use what works best in your specific situation. The important thing is that you record your hot flashes as *accurately* as possible.

RECORD YOUR "BASELINE" HOT FLASHES FOR ONE WEEK

A blank version of the Hot Flash Daily Diary is at the end of this chapter, in the appendix, and available at www.demoshealth .com/store/elkins-relief-from-hot-flashes-supplements. Feel free to print or make copies or use the ones at the end of each chapter as you follow the program. I know it will be tempting to get started right away with using the audio recordings and working through the program, but *please do not underestimate the importance of knowing your baseline hot flash information.*

Baseline
HOT FLASH DAILY DIARY

Date	Make a mark for each hot flash to indicate mild, moderate, severe, or very severe				Total # of Hot Flashes Today	NOTES (Use this space to record possible triggers or other information relating to trends you may notice about your hot flashes)
	MILD	MODE-RATE	SEVERE	VERY SEVERE		
MON / /	_____	_____	_____	_____		
TUES / /	_____	_____	_____	_____		
WEDS / /	_____	_____	_____	_____		
THURS / /	_____	_____	_____	_____		
FRI / /	_____	_____	_____	_____		
SAT / /	_____	_____	_____	_____		
SUN / /	_____	_____	_____	_____		
TOTALS						

Severity Descriptors

Mild	Lasts <5 minutes; uncomfortable warmth; mild discomfort; no need for action
Moderate	Up to 15 minutes; warm, clammy skin; increased heart rate; some sweating; agitated; embarrassed; use fan, remove clothes, etc.
Severe	Up to 20 minutes; very hot; increased heart rate; unusual sensation over skin; sweating; anxiety; embarrassment; activity interruption
Very severe	Up to 45 minutes; extreme heat; rolling perspiration; increased heart rate; nausea; extreme distress; difficulty functioning; need to take cold shower or hold ice on skin

Chapter 8

Identifying Your Hot Flash Triggers

s you collect your baseline data, which will give you a good approximation of how many hot flashes you are having each day and how severe they are, you may recognize some events, emotions, or activities that actually seem to contribute to, or "trigger," the onset of a hot flash.

Scientifically speaking, while the physiology of hot flashes is associated with a decrease in estrogen level or an increase in gonadotropin concentrations, the actual physiological mechanism of hot flashes is not known. While they may sometimes seem to occur spontaneously with no prior warning, it has also been reported that there are often "triggers" that precede hot flashes.

WHAT IS A HOT FLASH TRIGGER?

A hot flash trigger is anything that appears to precede a hot flash on a regular basis. Some who experience hot flashes report an aura just before the hot flash begins. Triggers may be termed as (1) external, (2) internal, or (3) learned (see the table on the next page).

EXTERNAL	INTERNAL	LEARNED
Temperature fluctuations	Anxiety	Entering a certain room
Alcohol	Stress	Applying make-up
Hot or spicy foods/beverages	Illness (i.e.: migraines, coughing)	Planning a dinner menu
Caffeine	Emotional situations	Getting ready for church

Some of the more common triggers identified by women experiencing hot flashes are:
- Stress/Anxiety
- Emotional situations
- Foods
- Drugs/Alcohol
- Environment/Activities

STRESS/ANXIETY

Psychological stress is often identified as a precursor to hot flashes. This stress may come from a host of factors, each as individual as you are from others. Making an attempt to identify the stressors that appear to preempt a hot flash could be helpful to you in a couple of ways.

1. The situation may be controllable. It may mean reducing stress by changing a situation, saying "no" to a new demand, or just taking time to relax.
2. If the stress cannot be reduced through a change in behavior, you will be able to use the tools you learn in this program to control the stress that can trigger a hot flash.

EMOTIONAL SITUATIONS

There are certain situations in which you may find that extreme emotions may precede a hot flash. In these cases, symptoms of the hot flash may even exacerbate the emotional feelings as you also feel embarrassment and discomfort relating to the hot flash.

FOODS

While certainly not limited to these, the foods most commonly attributed to triggering a hot flash are spicy foods, hot foods and beverages, and caffeine. As you begin to be more aware of when and how your hot flashes occur, you may notice that certain foods you eat or beverages you drink act as a precursor to your hot flashes. With this information, you may choose to alter some of your dietary habits as you proceed through the program.

DRUGS/ALCOHOL

Hot flashes have reportedly been associated with alcohol and certain medications, such as niacin. Niacin is sometimes prescribed to help raise the high-density lipoprotein, or HDL, for patients being treated for high cholesterol. This medication has potential side effects, one of the more common of which is hot flashes. Hot flashes generally occur within minutes of taking a niacin dose.

Alcohol consumption can also trigger hot flashes for some women. The mechanisms for alcohol-provoked hot flashes are complex, and sensitivity varies. However, it is known that alcohol causes vasodilation in the face and neck that can trigger a hot flash.

As she became aware of her triggers, Emily noticed that whenever she had a glass of wine (or two) this was *always* followed by a severe hot flash. While she didn't want to forego her wine with dinner altogether, she adapted her activity and used what she learned in the hypnotic relaxation therapy program to make a change. She reduced the amount of wine she had with dinner, and began using self-hypnosis when needed as she enjoyed her dinner.

ENVIRONMENT/ACTIVITIES

In some cases, environment may prompt a hot flash, especially when it is crowded, loud, or hot. You may also note that a certain activity, not normally associated with sweating, almost always precedes a hot flash.

For example, Emily reported that every morning as she was about to put on her makeup, she would have a hot flash. This was very frustrating for her as the sweat on her face caused a problem with putting on her makeup, sometimes even causing her to run late for her job. We talked about where and when she normally put on her makeup to see if there was anything that she could possibly do to change that activity from "a trigger to a hot flash" to simply "putting on makeup." Emily typically put her makeup on in the dressing area of her bathroom, a space shared with her husband, who was brushing his teeth or shaving at the same time. Above the dressing counter mirror were four high-wattage light bulbs. It was described as a "rush time" (which could also be called "stress time"). During our discussion, Emily decided to start putting her makeup on in her bedroom, seated at a small dressing table. She would do this alone and allow herself ample time so that she didn't feel crowded or rushed. At a later session, Emily reported that she had made the move to her bedroom for putting on her makeup. She stated that, "It gives me a special feeling... to have my own space that is quiet and uncrowded. I bought a lighted makeup mirror that doesn't get hot like the bathroom lights. I even play soft music while I put my makeup on, and if I feel [a hot flash] coming on, I take a moment to relax and imagine my cool place. I've still had hot flashes some, but they are not as often and not *nearly* as severe."

This is another example of how, once a trigger is identified, there may be behavioral changes that, when made in conjunction with the program, can help in reducing the frequency and, especially, the severity of hot flashes.

IDENTIFYING, THEN *CHANGING OR AVOIDING* YOUR HOT FLASH TRIGGERS

Once you have determined a relationship between your hot flashes and things that may seem to be associated with them, you will be able to use this awareness to supplement the program with some behavioral changes. For example, as you begin the hypnotic relaxation therapy program, you may happily realize that by giving up a glass of wine or doing without the extra hot salsa when eating at your favorite Mexican restaurant, you are having fewer hot flashes.

In Emily's case, she found it helpful to record some of the activities she was doing when she would have a hot flash. The following page contains is a sample Hot Flash Triggers form on which Emily recorded some of her potential triggers. As you look at what she recorded, you will notice that Emily has clearly identified stress, environmental temperature, and alcohol as potential triggers for her hot flashes. By seeing this pattern, she was able to look at the activities associated with the trigger and determine if she could make any changes that would affect the situation and possibly help with the hot flashes, as she did in the two examples given earlier.

This is a tool you may find helpful, or you may already be so attuned to your hot flashes that you are able to identify whether there seems to be a recurring or common denominator with regard to anything that may be considered a trigger. On the other hand, you may already know that there *does not* seem to be *any* rhyme or reason to your hot flashes. Each woman's experience with hot flashes is as individual and unique as the woman herself.

Following Emily's completed form noting the things that she noticed could trigger a hot flash for her, is a blank version of the Hot Flash Triggers log for your use if you feel it would be helpful. A blank Hot Flash Triggers log is also available in the appendix and at www.demoshealth.com/store/elkins-relief-from-hot-flashes-supplements.

Emily's
HOT FLASH TRIGGERS

POTENTIAL TRIGGER	ACTIVITY
Stress	Getting kids ready for vacation bible school
Stress	Watching granddaughter's softball game
Sleeping	Woke three times
Hot bathroom	Putting on makeup
Stress	Getting ready for work
Stress	Shopping
Sleeping	Woke three times
Temperature	Working in the garden
Stress	Trying to find my keys
Alcohol	Two glasses of wine
Sleep	Woke multiple times
Temperature	Putting on my makeup
Stress	Paying bills and balancing checkbook
Stress	Watching grandson's ball game
Sleep	Slept very badly; woke sweating many times

HOT FLASH TRIGGERS

POTENTIAL TRIGGER	ACTIVITY

Chapter 9

Assessing Your Sleep

D uring the menopausal transition, you can expect to experience a number of changes that will affect different areas of your life. Sleep problems have been identified among the most commonly reported menopause-specific symptoms. As you progress through this program, you will be asked to develop an awareness of your sleep patterns. You will be able to do this by completing a brief assessment prior to beginning your practice sessions. The assessment is called the "Baseline Sleep Rating Form" and is provided

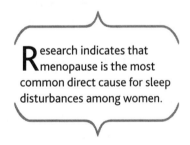

R esearch indicates that menopause is the most common direct cause for sleep disturbances among women.

at the end of this chapter. I believe you will see improvement in your sleep quality as you experience fewer hot flashes.

HOT FLASHES AND SLEEP

Sleep problems are very common during menopause. Research has shown that up to 50% of women report sleep difficulties. Further, the problem of poor sleep increases during menopause and up to 80% of women report changes in sleep postmenopause. While it is true that in the natural aging process, both men and women experience sleep disturbances, research has suggested that hot flashes are among the most common causes for disrupted sleep during the menopause transition.

You will possibly recognize many of these changes and symptoms in your own life, depending on where you are in the menopausal transition. Typically, hot flashes and night sweats occur more frequently during the perimenopausal stage and for younger women who have undergone surgical removal of ovaries or a treatment that inhibits the ability of the ovaries to produce hormones. It has been reported that the duration of hot flashes averages one to two years; however, in some cases hot flashes can last for five years or even for 10 or 20 years.

BASELINE AWARENESS OF SLEEP

While this book's primary objective is to equip you with the tools to help you to reduce or eliminate your hot flashes, you will see improvements in other areas of your life, such as your sleep quality.

The right amount of sleep each person needs to feel well-rested and able to function optimally varies from person to person based on a number of considerations, such as activity level, age, and an individual's life demands. For example, if a person is more physically active, they may need more sleep. The range of acceptable (healthy) sleep duration may vary among individuals from four to ten hours; however, the average for Americans is seven to eight hours per night. Please note the word *average*, as many people are well-rested with six hours (or less), and 10% to 15% need nine or more hours each day to feel well-rested.

As you begin this program, another important fact to consider is that sleep patterns change throughout our life span. However, while the number of hours may vary from person to person or life-stage to life-stage, the determining definition for good sleep quality is that you *feel rested and alert during the day.*

HOW IMPORTANT IS SLEEP?

Although research has shown that people with poor sleep quality, including insomnia, are capable of functioning quite well, those people (and perhaps you are included) find that things are harder to do and it requires more concentrated exertion to perform even the most routine tasks. They also express concern that they did not do as well as they would have expected or liked to do.

Your physical health may suffer because of sleepless nights. In animal studies, extreme long-term sleep disturbances have reportedly been shown to affect the immune system. Additionally, sleep loss may be associated with an increased psychological stress level.

Depending on where you are right now with your hot flashes, you may be asking yourself a variation of an age-old question—"Which came first: the sleepless nights or the night sweats?" As you move through this 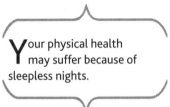 book, you may be able to answer this for yourself, or you may simply decide that it's as unanswerable as the original chicken/egg version. And to be honest, it does not matter. The important thing to remember is that you will be able to see improvement in how you feel as you reduce the frequency and severity of your hot flashes and improve your sleep quality.

ASSESSING YOUR SLEEP

The Sleep Rating Form will help you to see any changes in your quality of sleep over time. A blank form is provided at the end of this chapter, in the appendix, and at www.demoshealth.com/ store/elkins-relief-from-hot-flashes-supplements. You should complete this form prior to beginning your recorded hypnosis practice sessions, after the conclusion of your final practice session (approximately five weeks later), and again approximately six weeks after that. By completing this questionnaire prior to beginning your practice sessions, you will have a baseline point of reference you can compare your answers to on all subsequent questionnaires.

To begin, you will be asked to approximate how many hours of sleep you feel you have gotten each night during the previous week.

Then, you will rate ten statements about your sleep quality on a scale of 0 (not at all) to 10 (very much so).

Finally, you will establish your "sleep score" by adding the numbers you have circled. This score can then be compared to your score once you have completed five weeks of this program.

HOW WAS EMILY'S SLEEP?

The facing page shows a copy of Emily's completed baseline Sleep Rating Form, which indicates she was getting about four to five hours of sleep each night with considerable sleep disturbances.

Emily often felt very tired during the day as she went about her daily routine. She also reported difficulty concentrating on tasks, and would often "forget what [she] was doing."

RATE YOUR SLEEP

Please take a moment to complete the blank baseline "Sleep Rating Form" at the end of this chapter to get an idea of how you are sleeping. This will give you a good idea of how well you are sleeping!

MOVING FORWARD

Once you complete the Sleep Rating Form you will have a score that gives you an indication of your sleep quality. Moving forward then, to chapter 10, we will discuss a form that will help you determine to what degree hot flashes may affect your mood, your interpersonal relationships, and your overall quality of life. Completing these forms now will help you later on when you begin to track your progress!

Emily's Baseline
SLEEP RATING FORM

DATE: 7/29/xx

During the past week, about how many hours did you sleep each night on average? 4.5

Circle the number that best represents your agreement with the following comments regarding your sleep *during the past week.*

	Not at all									Very much so	
1. I was relaxed during my sleep.	0	1	2	③	4	5	6	7	8	9	10
2. I went to sleep quickly.	0	1	②	3	4	5	6	7	8	9	10
3. My sleep was good.	0	1	2	③	4	5	6	7	8	9	10
4. I awoke very few times during the night.	0	1	2	③	4	5	6	7	8	9	10
5. For my age, I felt like I got an adequate amount of sleep.	0	1	2	3	④	5	6	7	8	9	10
6. I was satisfied with my sleep.	0	1	2	③	4	5	6	7	8	9	10
7. My sleep met my expectations.	0	1	2	③	4	5	6	7	8	9	10
8. I was able to go to sleep without sleeping pills or drugs.	0	1	2	3	④	5	6	7	8	9	10
9. I stayed asleep most of the night.	0	①	2	3	4	5	6	7	8	9	10
10. I woke up feeling refreshed.	0	1	2	③	4	5	6	7	8	9	10

TOTAL SCORE: 29

("I slept well": 0 = not at all; 100 = very much so)

Baseline
SLEEP RATING FORM

DATE: _____

During the past week, about how many hours did you sleep each night on average? _____

Circle the number that best represents your agreement with the following comments regarding your sleep *during the past week.*

	Not at all									Very much so
1. I was relaxed during my sleep.	0	1	2	3	4	5	6	7	8	9	10
2. I went to sleep quickly.	0	1	2	3	4	5	6	7	8	9	10
3. My sleep was good.	0	1	2	3	4	5	6	7	8	9	10
4. I awoke very few times during the night.	0	1	2	3	4	5	6	7	8	9	10
5. For my age, I felt like I got an adequate amount of sleep.	0	1	2	3	4	5	6	7	8	9	10
6. I was satisfied with my sleep.	0	1	2	3	4	5	6	7	8	9	10
7. My sleep met my expectations.	0	1	2	3	4	5	6	7	8	9	10
8. I was able to go to sleep without sleeping pills or drugs.	0	1	2	3	4	5	6	7	8	9	10
9. I stayed asleep most of the night.	0	1	2	3	4	5	6	7	8	9	10
10. I woke up feeling refreshed.	0	1	2	3	4	5	6	7	8	9	10

TOTAL SCORE: _____

("I slept well": 0 = not at all; 100 = very much so)

Chapter 10

Rating the Interference of Your Hot Flashes on Your Mood, Relationships, and Quality of Life

W hen hot flashes are frequent they can interfere with daily activities and emotional well-being. As you prepare to begin this program, it is important that you are also aware of how hot flashes are affecting your everyday life.

In this chapter, I'll help you understand the ways hot flashes affect mood, relationships, and quality of life (QOL); help you to recognize these impacts in your own life; and provide you with a tool, the Hot Flash Related Daily Interference Scale (HFRDIS), to track QOL improvement as your hot flashes become less frequent and severe.

THE EFFECT OF HOT FLASHES ON MOOD

Hot flashes can have a significant effect on your mood. They can cause stress and irritability. The effect of hot flashes on mood can be direct or indirect. A direct effect is that the sweating and emotional arousal during a hot flash can lead to anxiety and irritability. An indirect effect is when hot flashes interfere with sleep; the resulting fatigue and decreased energy can contribute to stress. An increase in anxiety and stress can cause some women to experience more hot flashes. A six-year study of postmenopausal women found that anxiety was a strong predictor of an increase in hot flashes. Women who reported moderate anxiety levels were three times more likely to report hot flashes and those with high anxiety levels were *five times* more likely to report hot flashes.

In addition, a significant association has been reported between depressive symptoms and hot flashes. Women who are very depressed or having a lot of stress in their lives may have more hot flashes. It is noteworthy that in the studies of hypnotic relaxation for hot flashes, women, in fact, report a lessening of feelings of depression and anxiety as hot flashes become less frequent and sleep becomes better. These are additional benefits of using the *Relief from Hot Flashes* program.

Rating your mood will help you to notice that as your hot flashes decrease, your mood, anxiety, and stress levels will also improve.

THE EFFECT OF HOT FLASHES ON RELATIONSHIPS

Hot flashes can also impact your relationships with coworkers, classmates, family members, and friends or acquaintances. The physical characteristics of a hot flash may include hot skin, a red face, neck, or ears, and excessive sweating. Any one, and certainly a combination of more than one, of these symptoms could cause a disruption in your daily life, especially when it comes to relationships.

Relations with Others

The ability to enjoy close relationships can be disrupted when hot flashes cause anxiety, fatigue, or embarrassment.

Work

The onset of a hot flash at work may lead to embarrassment, feelings of distress, panic, and possibly even a decrease in work productivity as you work to maintain the relationships you have developed in your workplace.

Social Activities

Hot flashes can also affect your social activities as they can interfere with your enjoyment of going to parties, attending church, participating in social gatherings, or spending quality time spent with your family and friends.

Leisure Activities

Depending on your lifestyle, you may have noticed ways that hot flashes can interfere with things you do for fun or health. For example, hot flashes can occur when a person is exercising, playing tennis, attending an aerobics class, or going for walks in the evening. Some women avoid exercise for fear of triggering a hot flash.

Sex

One very important dynamic is that of sexual intimacy. With the onset of hot flashes, many women report that they experience night sweats so intensely that physical closeness and intimacy become unpleasant for them, resulting in a negative impact on their relationship with a romantic partner.

THE EFFECT OF HOT FLASHES ON QUALITY OF LIFE

QOL is a term used to explain your general well-being. In health care, QOL is defined as the perceived quality of one's daily life, or how much a person enjoys his or her life. QOL encompasses many aspects of your life including enjoyment of daily activities, social relationships, physical well-being, sleep, mood, and level of stress. Because hot flashes can have an impact on so many parts of your life, they can diminish your perceived QOL.

THE HOT FLASH RELATED DAILY INTERFERENCE SCALE

The HFRDIS is a brief 10-item questionnaire that asks you to rate the level of interference you perceive hot flashes to cause with different aspects of your life. A blank form is provided at the end of this chapter, in the appendix, and at www.demoshealth.com/store/elkins-relief-from-hot-flashes-supplements.

It will ask you to rate the how much hot flashes interfere with your work, social activities, leisure activities, sleep, mood, concentration, relations with others, sexuality, enjoyment of life, and overall QOL. Once you have selected a response from 0 (not at all) to 10 (very much so) for each item, you will then arrive at a total score by adding the numbers together, giving you a total score that will rate the statement "Hot flashes interfered with my life" on a scale of 0 (not at all) to 100 (very much so).

Complete this questionnaire prior to beginning your hypnotic relaxation therapy practice sessions and after you have completed the five-week program.

HOW DID EMILY RATE THE INTERFERENCE OF HOT FLASHES?

As Emily began the program, we discussed some of the areas of concern she had that were related to hot flash interference. For instance, she reported that hot flashes were a great source of embarrassment for her at work, especially in the classroom. Though Emily and I met during the summer months, she was truly bothered by her past (and what she feared would be future) experience with hot flashes as she taught her students. Emily's students were sixth and seventh graders, so certainly old enough to be aware that something was going on with her when she had a hot flash. She described a typical hot flash in the classroom as *extremely* interfering, and stated further:

"I'll be talking to the class, and suddenly I'll feel the hot flash as it begins. I immediately start feeling… what I guess could be described as 'panicky,' because I know what is about to happen, and I also know I have no hope of controlling it. So at this point, I lose my concentration on what I was teaching my class, and then, when my face becomes blood red and sweat starts pouring, the students lose their concentration as they start asking me if I'm 'alright.' It's very embarrassing, as I don't want to discuss menopause with a classroom of preteens. This can cause us to lose 20, and sometimes even more, minutes of valuable learning time, and I find that very distressing."

Emily also experienced times when she could not focus or concentrate on what she was doing. She reported having to "mentally walk myself through the steps" of many ordinary, everyday tasks in order to simply get through the day. For example, she said that most mornings, she will have to consciously tell herself to "pick up your toothbrush," "wet it," "put the toothpaste on," "brush," "rinse." Another area of concern for Emily was her interpersonal relationships. Emily was married to her high school sweetheart who worked for the postal service. She described him as "kind, quiet, laughs at all of my jokes, and eats my cooking, no matter how bad it is." She said that while they are still close, she sometimes feels moody and impatient with him. Regarding sexual intimacy, she said she just "cringes" at the thought of him touching her at times. When asked to explain, Emily said that when she had hot flashes, she did not want anything or anyone touching her. She was afraid that the sexual intimacy would bring on a hot flash and she could not stand the thought of having him touching her if one occurred. Emily assured me that the feelings she had were not in any way a reflection of her love for her husband. She loves him very much, and often feels guilty for having these negative feelings about him.

After her husband, the majority of her interpersonal relationships were with her children and grandchildren, coworkers, and friends from church. She reported that she had given up some activities altogether, such as her book club, because she did not want to have hot flashes in front of other members of the club.

Please take a look at how Emily completed the HFRDIS. Her ratings indicated that the hot flashes she was experiencing prior to beginning the program were interfering significantly with many areas of her life.

RATE THE INTERFERENCE OF HOT FLASHES ON YOUR MOOD, RELATIONSHIPS, AND QUALITY OF LIFE

After reviewing Emily's completed HFRDIS, please complete yours. You will be able to compare your scores about six weeks from now after you complete the *Relief from Hot Flashes* program.

MOVING FORWARD

This program follows a specific process with identifiable steps. As you move into chapter 11 and the section entitled "Hypnotic Relaxation Therapy: The Solution for Hot Flashes," you will be able to get an even better idea of what to expect from the program together with other important information to consider as you start your individual use of hypnotic relaxation therapy and the program in earnest.

Emily's Baseline
HOT FLASH RELATED DAILY
INTERFERENCE SCALE (HFRDIS)

DATE: 7/23/xx

Circle the number that best describes how much hot flashes have interfered with each aspect of your life *during the past week*.

	Not at all										Very much so
1. Work (work outside the home and house work)	0	1	2	3	4	5	6	7	8	9	(10)
2. Social activities (time spent with family, friends, etc.)	0	1	2	3	4	5	6	(7)	8	9	10
3. Leisure activities (time spent relaxing, doing hobbies, etc.)	0	1	2	3	4	5	(6)	7	8	9	10
4. Sleep	0	1	2	3	4	5	6	7	8	9	(10)
5. Mood	0	1	2	3	4	5	6	7	8	(9)	10
6. Concentration	0	1	2	3	4	5	6	7	8	9	(10)
7. Relations with others	0	1	2	3	4	5	6	7	(8)	9	10
8. Sexuality	0	1	2	3	4	5	6	7	8	(9)	10
9. Enjoyment of life	0	1	2	3	4	5	6	7	(8)	9	10
10. Overall quality of life	0	1	2	3	4	5	6	7	8	(9)	10

TOTAL SCORE: ___86___

("Hot flashes interfered with my life": 0 = not at all; 100 = very much so)

Baseline
HOT FLASH RELATED DAILY
INTERFERENCE SCALE (HFRDIS)

DATE: _____

Circle the number that best describes how much hot flashes have interfered with each aspect of your life *during the past week*.

	Not at all										Very much so
1. Work (work outside the home and house work)	0	1	2	3	4	5	6	7	8	9	10
2. Social activities (time spent with family, friends, etc.)	0	1	2	3	4	5	6	7	8	9	10
3. Leisure activities (time spent relaxing, doing hobbies, etc.)	0	1	2	3	4	5	6	7	8	9	10
4. Sleep	0	1	2	3	4	5	6	7	8	9	10
5. Mood	0	1	2	3	4	5	6	7	8	9	10
6. Concentration	0	1	2	3	4	5	6	7	8	9	10
7. Relations with others	0	1	2	3	4	5	6	7	8	9	10
8. Sexuality	0	1	2	3	4	5	6	7	8	9	10
9. Enjoyment of life	0	1	2	3	4	5	6	7	8	9	10
10. Overall quality of life	0	1	2	3	4	5	6	7	8	9	10

TOTAL SCORE: _____

("Hot flashes interfered with my life": 0 = not at all; 100 = very much so)

HYPNOTIC RELAXATION THERAPY: THE SOLUTION FOR HOT FLASHES

Chapter 11

Hypnotic Relaxation Therapy: What Happens

You have learned how to use the Hot Flash Daily Diary and have an awareness of the frequency and severity of your hot flashes. In addition, you now have a good idea of your sleep quality and how hot flashes affect and interfere with your daily activities. As you begin your practice of hypnotic relaxation therapy it will be important for you to continue to maintain your Hot Flash Daily Diary. In this chapter I will provide you with a more complete walk-through of the process before you begin the actual program so you will know more specifically what to expect and a few best practices to keep in mind as you begin the program in earnest with the next chapter.

THE PROCESS OF HYPNOTIC RELAXATION

The process of hypnotic relaxation induction follows several simple steps. These steps can be achieved in different ways, but by having an idea of this process you will have an easier time of learning how to make it work best for you.

When you practice hypnotic relaxation you should be sitting in a comfortable chair with good support for your head, neck, and shoulders. If you prefer to lie down on a bed or floor, that is fine. Whatever you prefer is OK.

The steps in the process are:

Focusing Your Attention

This is the beginning of a hypnotic induction. You will be directed to focus your attention on a spot, an object, or an idea.

Eye Closure

Suggestions are then given for you to close your eyes. This helps to block out external stimuli and for you to be more aware of your own internal feelings and responses. Internal feelings associated with breathing are one example of the shift toward relaxation and a hypnotic state.

Achieving Hypnotic Relaxation

You will then hear suggestions for relaxation. There are physiological changes that occur with deep therapeutic relaxation. The hypnotic relaxation is both physical and mental. The mental relaxation leads to a deep emotional relaxation.

Physical Relaxation

Physical relaxation refers to the degree to which you are able to allow your body to relax. To help you understand relaxation I need to say a few words about the autonomic nervous system or ANS. The ANS is that part of our nervous system in which the brain and nerves react automatically. The ANS is divided into two parts: the sympathetic and the parasympathetic nervous systems.

The sympathetic nervous system is activated when we feel stress. The stress can be something that happens to us or simply from our own thoughts. However, when we feel stressed, the sympathetic nervous system causes muscles to tense and the body to become more tensed in general. This reaction occurs when we are worried, angry, or just dealing with daily activities. The tension can be, and often is, outside our conscious awareness.

The parasympathetic nervous system works in the opposite direction. It becomes activated when we become deeply relaxed. With physical relaxation there are a variety of changes that occur:

- Heart rate decreases
- Muscles relax
- Blood pressure decreases
- Breathing becomes slower and calmer
- Body temperature changes
- Metabolism is more relaxed

There are many benefits associated with these changes that are sometimes called the *relaxation response*. As therapeutic relaxation occurs, the parasympathetic nervous system is activated and this can give way to a greater sense of mental and emotional relaxation and calmness.

Mental and Emotional Relaxation

For many purposes, mental and emotional relaxation is even more important than physical relaxation. It is a feeling of calmness and a feeling of control. Calm thoughts and images occur and there is a general sense of well-being. As mental-emotional relaxation is achieved, worries and concerns are set aside for a brief period of time. Mental and emotional relaxation is associated with subjective changes such as:

> As mental–emotional relaxation is achieved, worries and concerns are set aside for a brief period of time.

- Calm thoughts
- Peaceful feelings
- External sounds and events can be ignored
- Observation of self
- Effortless relaxation responses
- Awareness of mental images

There is an inner feeling of peacefulness. With the mental and emotional relaxation we are able to begin to observe our thoughts and reactions. It seems to occur automatically and without much conscious effort. When it is achieved, you begin to drift into a hypnotic state.

Hypnotic State

The hypnotic state has been described as an "altered state of consciousness" and a state of concentration. There is a shift toward greater awareness of your own internal images and thoughts. In a hypnotic state you are more receptive to positive therapeutic hypnotic suggestions.

At the beginning of a hypnotic induction, during the "focus your attention" step, your focus is on some external object; then your focus turns toward an awareness of your breathing, feelings, and thoughts. As a hypnotic state is achieved, you reduce critical and judgmental thinking; you become aware of inner images; you begin to respond to those images as your reality; and you are more receptive to therapeutic suggestions.

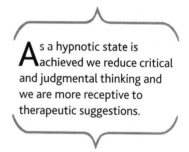

As a hypnotic state is achieved we reduce critical and judgmental thinking and we are more receptive to therapeutic suggestions.

With practice you can improve your ability to achieve a deeper level of hypnotic relaxation. It is sometimes helpful to think of the depth of hypnotic relaxation as proceeding through different stages. There are five stages that you will likely experience in varying degrees.

- **Alert state:** This is simply where you begin. It is everyday alertness.
- **Hypnodial stage:** This stage refers to your preparation for hypnotic relaxation. As you focus your attention and close your eyes you will notice a more relaxed feeling. You are not in a hypnotic state at that point, but it is a precursor to the hypnotic state.
- **Light stage:** Here you will begin to experience deeper relaxation. You may notice your breathing becoming slower, feelings of heaviness in your arms and legs, and you begin to see vague images.

- **Medium stage:** In this stage, there are changes in sensations. You may notice a rocking sensation or a feeling of even deeper relaxation.
- **Deep stage:** There is a more profound response to suggestions in the deep stage of hypnotic relaxation. For example, if suggestions for coolness are given, you may feel cold and experience chill bumps. Mental images are most vivid.

Mental Imagery

In a hypnotic state, mental images are experienced as real even if you are aware that they are images. This is similar to a vivid dream or intense daydreaming. As mental images are suggested, it is possible to become so absorbed in experiencing those images that your thoughts, feelings, and reactions reflect that you experience them as "real." When you listen to the audio recordings included with this book, you will hear suggestions for mental imagery that will include images of being in a safe place where you feel calm and cool.

Safe Place Imagery

In order to have a feeling of "letting go" and to achieve the deepest level of relaxation, it is essential to feel safe. Therefore, hypnotic relaxation suggestions include mental imagery for a place where you feel very safe and secure. This can be imagery for being in a garden, on vacation, or even at home. It is a place that is often very personal, and the specific imagery can be intensified by focusing on the details of the imagined place and surroundings.

Calmness

You will be asked to think about places and times where you felt very calm and relaxed. Calmness is a subjective feeling, and when it is achieved in a hypnotic relaxation session it can continue beyond the session and throughout the day.

Coolness

Hot flashes are believed to be related to a dysfunction in the thermoregulatory system. It is logical to assume that if the brain perceives coolness there is no need for a hot flash. This is essential to controlling hot flashes. I suggest mental images that are strongly associated with coolness. This could include feeling a cool breeze, snow, a shower, or even the coolness from an air conditioner. As you hold these images firmly, you experience the physical and emotional feelings associated with the images. With this program of hypnotic relaxation, you will begin to learn the specific kinds of images for coolness that work best for you.

Posthypnotic Suggestion

Posthypnotic suggestions are those that reference effects that continue after the hypnotic relaxation session is over. In this case it will include suggestions for increased control and reduction of hot flashes.

Alerting

After goals are accomplished and a session of hypnotic relaxation comes to an end, you will be prompted to return to conscious alertness. During a session of hypnotic relaxation you are aware of your surroundings, but they are more or less in the background of your awareness. With suggestions for alertness you become more aware of the present time and place and these things then move into the foreground of your awareness. Conscious alertness may be achieved by counting silently to yourself or simply by opening your eyes. You will find what is most comfortable for you.

In addition, there are several things that you can do to make sure you make the most of your practice of hypnotic relaxation. These key things for your successful practice will now be summarized.

MAKE SUFFICIENT TIME TO PRACTICE

It is essential to your success that you make time to practice. In this program, you should plan to practice one or more times per day for about 25 to 30 minutes for each practice session. You will need to make arrangements so that you are not disturbed or interrupted during your practice times. That can mean letting family members know that you are going to practice, putting pets in another room, and having a quiet place for your practice session. For some people, simply finding such protected time can be challenging, so more will be said about this in later chapters. However, to summarize:

- In the first five weeks set aside 25 to 30 minutes to practice hypnotic relaxation one or more times a day
- Find a quiet place
- Ask that you not be interrupted during your practice time

APPROACH WITH CONFIDENCE

It is important for you to have a feeling of confidence in yourself and in your ability to use hypnotic relaxation. This is part of the reason I have presented so much information on the past research on this program for treatment of hot flashes. With this increased knowledge you can be more confident in knowing that there is substantial evidence for its effectiveness. Also, as you maintain a daily diary to record your hot flashes you will see them decline. And as you have your own personal experience of being able to reduce your hot flashes, your self-confidence will increase, and so will the effectiveness of the program.

BELIEVE IN YOUR HYPNOTIC ABILITIES

There is considerable research to indicate that people vary in their hypnotic ability; however, everyone has some degree of hypnotic abilities, or "hypnotizability." Some people are in a very low range and some have a very high hypnotic ability. The vast majority of us are in the middle. The best way to think of hypnotic abilities is as a talent or an innate ability. For example, some people have a great deal of talent and can learn to play a new musical instrument or sing a song with ease. Other people, myself included, would need to practice quite a bit to learn to play music. But most people will develop some ability to play music if given time and the right training. The same is true for hypnotic ability.

There is considerable research to indicate that people vary in their hypnotic ability; however, everyone has some degree of hypnotic abilities, or "hypnotizability."

There is no way to know exactly what your hypnotic ability or talent is without beginning a hypnotic induction. There are some scales that measure hypnotizability; however, all of those measures involve a hypnotic induction and then seeing how well a person responds to suggestions. Once you complete a hypnotic induction using the audio recordings you will be able to estimate for yourself how well you were able to respond. You may think of the depth of hypnotic relaxation response on a 0–100 scale, where "0" represents a state of complete alertness and "100" represents the deepest level possible. In using such a scale, the things you will want to be aware of and assess are how deeply relaxed you feel, how vivid the mental imagery is experienced, and, of course, how quickly the hot flashes become less frequent and less severe.

If you are blessed with a high degree of hypnotic ability it is likely that you will be able to achieve a deeply relaxed state and reduce your hot flashes quickly. Many people experience a significant reduction after a week or two of daily practice. On the other hand, if you are in the lower range of hypnotic ability, it may take you a bit longer and require more practice to get the same result. This is one case where persistence pays off! Do not become discouraged if it takes you a few weeks to make your hot flashes decrease. In previous studies virtually all patients were able to reduce their hot flashes over time, and I'm confident you will, too.

You are now ready to begin your first week of learning the practice of hypnotic relaxation.

Chapter 12

Week 1: Starting Your Practice

The audio files: *Hypnotic Relaxation for Hot Flashes-Mountain Imagery* **and** *Hypnotic Relaxation for Hot Flashes-Lake Imagery* **accompany this chapter.**[*]

A t this point you have gained considerable knowledge about hot flashes and hypnotic relaxation therapy. You have all of the tools you need to begin and four completed forms recording your baseline measurements for your hot flashes, triggers, sleep, and quality of life. In this chapter, I will guide you into your first practice session using the audio recordings.

The practice of hypnotic relaxation is very effective, but it does require time and effort. The benefit is worth it, so let's get into the program!

WEEK 1

The goal for this week is for you to develop familiarity with the program, establish a routine of daily practice, and begin to identify what works best for you. There are two audio recordings available for use in the first week because preferences for mental imagery vary: *Hypnotic Relaxation Therapy for Hot Flashes-Mountain Imagery* or *Hypnotic Relaxation Therapy for Hot Flashes-Lake Imagery*. You may choose only

* To access these files, visit www.demoshealth.com/store/elkins-relief-from-hot-flashes-supplements

one or use them both alternately over the next seven days. You may find that you prefer to imagine being near a beautiful lake to being in the mountains. It is entirely up to you. Each recording follows the same process. Let's review that now so you'll know what to expect.

WHAT TO EXPECT ON THE AUDIO RECORDINGS

On the recordings, you will hear my voice as you are asked to focus your attention by looking at a spot on the wall or your selected point of focus. I will then give you suggestions to become relaxed and to drift into a hypnotic state where you can respond to suggestions.

There is nothing you need to do and nothing you need to try to do. Just allow yourself to respond in whatever way you respond. The recordings proceed in the stages described earlier.

Focus of Attention

You will be directed to focus your attention on a focal point (spot, sticker, small object, etc.) on the wall or ceiling. As you concentrate, begin to feel more relaxed. Concentrate intensely so that other things begin to fade into the background. Take a deep breath of air, hold, and as you exhale become more relaxed.

Eye Closure

You will then be asked to take another breath of air and, as you exhale, allow your eyelids to close. You may notice that your eyelids feel heavy and that you already begin to feel more relaxed.

Achieving Hypnotic Relaxation

The suggestions for relaxation involve noticing a "wave of relaxation" that spreads from the top of your head to the bottom of your feet. This relaxation can become deeper as I count the numbers from 1 to 20.

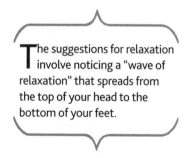

The suggestions for relaxation involve noticing a "wave of relaxation" that spreads from the top of your head to the bottom of your feet.

With each number I'll give suggestions that will prompt you to become more relaxed—physically, mentally, and emotionally.

As you respond to these suggestions you may notice that my voice seems more in the background or that you have a feeling of lightness or floating. Some people become so relaxed that they feel their arms and legs become heavy. Whatever you notice is part of your overall experience of hypnotic relaxation.

Mental Imagery

Now you will be prompted to experience mental imagery for coolness. Depending on which audio recording you choose, you will hear me describe the imagery of either walking down a mountain path on a cool day or sitting near a lake and feeling coolness. You will be given suggestions to experience a cool breeze, cool mountain air, a cool mist, and/or to visualize snow around you. You may find that you become aware of other images from your subconscious that are related to relaxation and coolness.

Posthypnotic Suggestions

Suggestions will be given for additional positive changes to occur in the weeks ahead—these will include better sleep, feeling less stress, and reducing frequency and severity of hot flashes. All will be given in a positive manner, with the expectation of these changes occurring in the near future. You will also be given suggestions for continued practice of hypnotic relaxation.

Alerting

Suggestions will be given for returning to conscious alertness. This will be done by presenting some numbers with the suggestion that each number can serve as a cue to return to conscious alertness. You may return to alertness or you may drift off into sleep. It is your choice and in your control. If you drift into sleep you will awaken naturally and feel refreshed.

TEN STEPS TO SUCCESSFUL PRACTICE

There are ten steps to successful practice of hypnotic relaxation therapy for hot flashes. With each practice session, review these steps so that they become automatic for you and a natural part of your routine as you progress through this program.

**Ten Steps to Successful Practice of
Hypnotic Relaxation for Hot Flashes**

1. Find a quiet place to practice.
2. Make arrangements to avoid interruptions.
3. Do not engage in any other activity during your practice time.
4. Rate your level of relaxation before practice and after.
5. Focus your attention on the audio recording.
6. Adopt an attitude of "letting go" and calmness.
7. Notice relaxation.
8. Notice mental images and feelings of coolness.
9. Have an awareness of when and how to practice that works best for you.
10. Maintain your Hot Flash Daily Diary.

LET'S BEGIN

Find a place that is relatively quiet. You may want to use headphones while you practice—they may be helpful in blocking out unwanted sounds. Make arrangements to not be disturbed during your practice time. The audio recording is about 30 minutes long, so you need at least that amount of time to be "protected time" with no interruptions. Do not engage in any other activity while you practice. You should not read, watch television, drive a car, or engage in *any* other activity.

Take a moment to rate your level of relaxation on a scale of 0–10, with "0" representing "no relaxation at all" and "10" representing "as relaxed as I possibly could be."

0------1------2------3------4------5------6------7------8------9------10

No relaxation at all   As relaxed as I possibly could be

Now, lie down or sit in a chair with good support for your head, neck, and shoulders. As you focus on the audio recording, adopt an attitude of "letting go" and calmness. As you become more relaxed, notice the images of coolness that will be suggested to you.

Select the recording that you most associate with coolness and comfort, either *Hypnotic Relaxation Therapy for Hot Flashes-Mountain Imagery* or *Hypnotic Relaxation Therapy for Hot Flashes-Lake Imagery*, press play, and begin.

POSTSESSION

Upon completion of your hypnotic relaxation session please rate your level of relaxation again.

0------1------2------3------4------5------6------7------8------9------10

No relaxation at all   As relaxed as I possibly could be

Also, once you have completed your first practice session, jot down a few notes regarding your experience. You may find it helpful to complete this after each practice session as a tool to help you identify personal and individual preferences for imagery. As you reflect on your completed practice session, simply make a few notes regarding the following questions.

What were you most aware of when you opened your eyes after listening to the audio recording?

_____

_____

Which part of the audio recording did you like the best?

_____

_____

Were there some suggestions that seemed to help you relax the most?

_____

_____

Did you experience some aspects of the mental images (mountains, lake, coolness) that were suggested?

_____

_____

Did you notice any other images or memories that helped you to become relaxed and find coolness?

_____

_____

IN THE WEEK AHEAD

Plan to Practice with the First Week's Audio Recording at Least Once Per Day

You may find that you have the best results by practicing in the morning, middle of the day, or in the evening. Some people find that using the recording at night, right before going to sleep, helps with going to sleep quicker, promotes more restful sleep, and decreases night sweats. At least once each day practice with either *Hypnotic Relaxation Therapy for Hot Flashes-Mountain Imagery* or *Hypnotic Relaxation Therapy for Hot Flashes-Lake Imagery.*

Maintain Your Hot Flash Daily Diary

You will be able to compare your progress from week to week. It is generally expected that after the first week of practice with the audio recordings you will see the number and severity of hot flashes decrease by as much as 30%.

At the end of this chapter you will find a blank Hot Flash Daily Diary for Week 1.

Track Your Triggers

Note situations where you tend to have hot flashes. Examples are when hot flashes occur in stressful situations, at work, after eating or drinking hot foods, alcohol use, and so on. Noting these things and maintaining your Hot Flash Daily Diary can help guide your practice because it can give you some indications of when, how, and how often to practice hypnotic relaxation therapy. For example, if you tend to have more hot flashes in stressful situations, you may want to use hypnotic relaxation prior to those situations.

At the end of this chapter you will find a blank Hot Flash Triggers form.

Complete a Hypnotic Relaxation Practice Checklist

At the end of this chapter you will find a blank Hypnotic Relaxation Practice Checklist for Week 1. It is important to record your practice of hypnotic relaxation each week so you can look back and see how often you have practiced on a weekly basis and how effective you have been in achieving relaxation. This information can help you determine what works best for you as you proceed through each week of the program.

Best wishes for a great week!

Go to the appendix or www.demoshealth.com/store/elkins-relief-from-hot-flashes-supplements to access additional blank copies of the:
Hot Flash Daily Diary
Hot Flash Triggers form
Hypnotic Relaxation Practice Checklist

Week 1
HOT FLASH DAILY DIARY

| Date | Make a mark for each hot flash to indicate mild, moderate, severe, or very severe | | | | Total # of Hot Flashes Today | NOTES (Use this space to record possible triggers or other information relating to trends you may notice about your hot flashes) |
	MILD	MODE-RATE	SEVERE	VERY SEVERE		
MON / /	_____	_____	_____	_____		
TUES / /	_____	_____	_____	_____		
WEDS / /	_____	_____	_____	_____		
THURS / /	_____	_____	_____	_____		
FRI / /	_____	_____	_____	_____		
SAT / /	_____	_____	_____	_____		
SUN / /	_____	_____	_____	_____		
TOTALS						

Severity Descriptors

Mild	Lasts <5 minutes; uncomfortable warmth; mild discomfort; no need for action
Moderate	Up to 15 minutes; warm, clammy skin; increased heart rate; some sweating; agitated; embarrassed; use fan, remove clothes, etc.
Severe	Up to 20 minutes; very hot; increased heart rate; unusual sensation over skin; sweating; anxiety; embarrassment; activity interruption
Very severe	Up to 45 minutes; extreme heat; rolling perspiration; increased heart rate; nausea; extreme distress; difficulty functioning; need to take cold shower or hold ice on skin

WEEK 1 HOT FLASH TRIGGERS

POTENTIAL TRIGGER	ACTIVITY

Week 1
HYPNOTIC RELAXATION
PRACTICE CHECKLIST

DATE: _____

Week #: ○ 1   ○ 2   ○ 3   ○ 4   ○ 5

1. *During the past week,* how often have you practiced hypnotic relaxation with the audio recording?

Daily (seven times per week) or more	☐
Three to six times per week	☐
One to two times per week	☐
None	☐

2. Please rate your average relaxation before hypnotic relaxation (presession average):

0	1	2	3	4	5	6	7	8	9	10
No relaxation										Extremely relaxed

3. Please rate your average relaxation after hypnotic relaxation (postsession average):

0	1	2	3	4	5	6	7	8	9	10
No relaxation										Extremely relaxed

Chapter 13

Week 2: Individualizing Your Practice

The audio file entitled *Individualizing Hypnotic Relaxation for Hot Flashes* accompanies this chapter.*

Congratulations! You have completed your first week of hypnotic relaxation practice. The audio recordings you used included mental imagery and suggestions for either walking along a mountain path or sitting near a lake. These images are associated with coolness and toward achieving regulation of body temperature, reduction of stress, and reduction of hot flashes. You may have found that one of the recordings works great for you and you may stay with that audio recording. However, you may make even more progress by finding some mental imagery that is individualized to you personally. This personalization can be built from your memories of relaxation and coolness and past experience. In this chapter, I will show you how to individualize your practice. But first, let's review your progress.

REVIEW YOUR WEEK 1 HOT FLASH DAILY DIARY AND CALCULATE YOUR HOT FLASH SCORE

Review your Hot Flash Daily Diary for the past week to see how you are doing after one week of practice of hypnotic relaxation therapy for reducing hot flashes. You will also want to calculate your hot flash score for this past week. Remember that your hot flash score represents a combination of the frequency and severity of your hot flashes for the week. Using the severity point values, take a moment now to calculate your Week 1 hot flash score.

- one point for a **mild** hot flash
- two points for a **moderate** hot flash
- three points for a **severe** hot flash
- four points for a **very severe** hot flash

Add up the number of hot flashes that you had for each category of severity rating.

Mild: Number of mild hot flashes multiplied times 1 = _____

Moderate: Number of moderate hot flashes multiplied times 2 = _____

Severe: Number of severe hot flashes multiplied times 3 = _____

Very Severe: Number of very severe hot flashes multiplied times 4 = _____

Add up the total to get your total hot flash score for the week = _____

Now that you have your hot flash score for the week, you can determine the percentage of reduction of your hot flashes in comparison to your baseline hot flash score. This is very useful because it will give you the information you need to very clearly determine how well you are doing and if there is anything you need to change to achieve significant reductions in hot flashes each week.

HOW TO CALCULATE THE PERCENTAGE REDUCTION IN HOT FLASH SCORE IN COMPARION TO YOUR BASELINE

It is important to be able to know how much your hot flash scores are decreasing each week. This can be done by a calculation of the percentage of change in hot flash scores in comparison to your baseline hot flash score. To calculate this percentage, follow the steps below.

Subtract the current week's hot flash score from your baseline hot flash score.

_____ Baseline hot flash score

− _____ Weekly hot flash score

= _____ Difference

Divide the difference by the baseline hot flash score.

_____ Difference

/ _____ Baseline hot flash score

= _____ Quotient

Multiply the quotient times 100 to determine the percentage of decrease.

_____ Quotient

× _____ 100

= _____ %

Here are three specific things to look for:

- Did the number of hot flashes decrease from the previous week?
- Is there a shift from severe/very severe toward mild/moderate in the severity rating of hot flashes?
- How does your hot flash score for this week compare to your baseline hot flash score?
- If your hot flash score decreased by 20% to 30% this past week, then you are perfectly on course with your program!

As an example, we can take a look at Emily's hot flash score and her percentage reduction for the week.

HOW DID EMILY DO?

Emily's Hot Flash Score

As you review Emily's Week 1 Hot Flash Daily Diary, you can see that her hot flashes are less frequent; however, there does not yet seem to be much change in the severity.

Emily's Week 1 hot flash score is shown below:

Mild:	7 hot flashes	× 1 = 7
Moderate:	14 hot flashes	× 2 = 28
Severe:	13 hot flashes	× 3 = 39
Very severe:	9 hot flashes	× 4 = 36

110 = Emily's Week 1
Hot Flash Score

Emily's Hot Flash Score Reduction Percentage

Step 1: Subtract the current week's hot flash score from the baseline hot flash score.

146   Emily's baseline hot flash score

−110   Emily's Week 1 hot flash score

36   Difference

Step 2: Divide the difference by the baseline hot flash score.

$36/146 = .25$

Step 3: Multiply the quotient times 100 to determine the percentage of decrease.

$.25 \times 100 = 25\%$

You can see that Emily's hot flashes decreased by 25%. This is consistent with what would be expected after the first week of the program.

Emily's Week 1
HOT FLASH DAILY DIARY

| Date | Make a mark for each hot flash to indicate mild, moderate, severe, or very severe | | | | Total # of Hot Flashes Today | NOTES (Use this space to record possible triggers or other information relating to trends you may notice about your hot flashes) |
	MILD	MODE-RATE	SEVERE	VERY SEVERE		
MON 7/30/xx	I	II	III	I	7	Stress 1X with night sweats
TUES 7/31/xx	I	II	II	II	7	Stress; makeup Woke 1X with sweats
WEDS 8/1/xx	II	II	I	I	6	Stress; worries Spicy foods/alcohol—had Mexican food w/margarita
THURS 8/2/xx	I	I	II	II	6	Stress; shopping Woke 2X's with night sweats
FRI 8/3/xx		III	I	II	6	Stress; alcohol: wine Woke 2X's with sweats
SAT 8/4/xx	I	II	I	I	5	Stress: attended funeral Makeup Woke 2X's with night sweats
SUN 8/5/xx	I	II	III		6	Stress; preparing for club presentation; alcohol-wine Woke 1X with night sweats
TOTALS	7	14	13	9	43	

Severity Descriptors

Mild	Lasts <5 min; uncomfortable warmth; mild discomfort; no need for action
Moderate	Up to 15 min; warm, clammy skin; increased heart rate; some sweating; agitated; embarrassed; use fan, remove clothes, etc.
Severe	Up to 20 min; very hot; increased heart rate; unusual sensation over skin; sweating; anxiety; embarrassment; activity interruption
Very severe	Up to 45 min; extreme heat; rolling perspiration; increased heart rate; nausea; extreme distress; difficulty functioning; need to take cold shower or hold ice on skin

REVIEW YOUR HYNPOTIC RELAXATION PRACTICE CHECKLIST AND TRIGGERS

Now, take a moment to look over your Hypnotic Relaxation Practice Checklist for the past week. Notice how many times you were able to practice. As you review the checklist, reflect on the exact time you practiced each day and if you missed any days. Did you practice more in the middle of the day or at night? Were you lying down or sitting up when you practiced? Did you experience any interruptions or were you undisturbed during your practice times? Does your average rating of relaxation show that you became more relaxed after a practice session?

Also, review your form for recording any triggers for hot flashes. Did you notice anything that triggered any hot flashes for you such as spicy foods, being in a hot room, or any specific stresses? Are there things you can do to eliminate or avoid these triggers? Make a mental note of any changes you believe you may need to make in the week ahead.

If you were able to decrease your hot flashes by 20% to 30%, there is probably nothing you need to change. If your hot flashes decreased by only 15% or less, then you should consider making some changes based on when and how frequently you practice hypnotic relaxation; you may need to practice more frequently. If you are having night sweats, you may need to practice at night before going to sleep. A careful review of the Hot Flash Daily Diary in conjunction with the checklist can help guide your practice in the week ahead.

EMILY'S WEEK 1 HYPNOTIC RELAXATION PRACTICE CHECKLIST

Now, let's take a look at Emily's Hypnotic Relaxation Practice Checklist to see how she did with daily practice. You can see that she practiced at least once per day and reported to me in our session that, on a couple of days, she practiced twice.

Emily's Week 1
HYPNOTIC RELAXATION
PRACTICE CHECKLIST

DATE: 8/5/xx

Week #:   ☒ 1   ○ 2   ○ 3   ○ 4   ○ 5

1. *During the past week, how often have you practiced hypnotic relaxation with the audio recording?*

   Daily (7 times per week) or more   ☒

   Three to six times per week   ☐

   One to two times per week   ☐

   None   ☐

2. Please rate your average relaxation before hypnotic relaxation (presession average):

   0   1   2   ③   4   5   6   7   8   9   10

   No   Extremely
   relaxation   relaxed

3. Please rate your average relaxation after hypnotic relaxation (postsession average):

   0   1   2   3   4   5   6   ⑦   8   9   10

   No   Extremely
   relaxation   relaxed

STARTING WEEK 2

This next week you will learn about individualization in your practice of hypnotic relaxation therapy. Individualization is the process of finding your own personal mental imagery for relaxation and coolness. This is achieved by reflecting on your own personal memories of such feelings. For example, you may recall a time while on vacation where you felt especially calm and relaxed while at the beach on a cool evening. Individualized images may occur to you spontaneously while practicing hypnotic relaxation, or you may be able to identify some personal images by reflecting on your experience.

Some questions that may help you identify the times and places that could best help with your hypnotic relaxation are:

- Do you recall a time when you felt especially relaxed and cool?
- If you could go on vacation to a place that is safe, relaxing, and cool, where would that be?
- What sensations do you notice when you feel calm and cool? Does that remind you of some other time in your life when you felt similar sensations of coolness?
- What makes you feel safe, pleasant, and relaxed?
- What experiences do you recall of feeling coolness (such as standing in front of an air conditioner, standing under a cool shower, swimming in a cool swimming pool, walking outside during a cool evening)?
- Can you imagine hot flashes "flowing out of your body" as you feel cool and relaxed?
- What type of suggestions help you to feel most cool and relaxed?

In response to the above questions, Emily identified a time when she was on vacation visiting her family in Michigan. She described staying at a vacation house near a lake and recalled walking from the back porch, down a hill, and to the lake to watch a sunset. Emily's description was rich in details of images, feelings, sensations of coolness, relaxation, and positive emotions that she could later visualize:

> *"I recall a time about 7:00 in the evening, standing on the back porch, looking down at the lake. I can see the water is very blue and still. There are lawn chairs near the bank of the lake and I can see my family there. I see my husband, my two children, and other members of my family. They are happy and they are talking. The grass is very green and I am barefoot. As I step onto the grass I notice that it is cool on my feet. I feel happy and relaxed. As I walk down to the lake, I can see the colors of the sky as the sun is setting. There are orange and blue and yellow colors, and a few clouds across the sky. I notice the coolness of the grass and there is a cool breeze in the air. I can feel the cool breeze across my face and neck. It feels good. As I reach the lake, I am greeted by my family; they are happy to see me. I feel loved and I see people that I love. As I sit in the lawn chair, I notice that the aluminum arms of the chair are cool. As I sit back, I relax. The sun is setting and I can feel the cool air blowing in from the lake."*

Take a moment now to write down your own personal mental images for relaxation and coolness. In the audio recording for this week, I will prompt you to use these images during your practice.

Notes on Individual Mental Imagery for Relaxation and Coolness:

_____

_____

_____

_____

_____

WHAT TO EXPECT ON THE AUDIO RECORDING

You will find the audio recording for this week to be similar to the previous ones. The overall process is now familiar to you. A difference is that in this audio recording of hypnotic relaxation there will be an indication for you to visualize your own personal imagery for relaxation and coolness noted above.

Focus of Attention

You will again be directed to focus your attention on a specific point. As you concentrate, I will suggest that you begin to feel more relaxed; then that other things begin to fade into the background. Finally, I will ask you to take a deep breath of air, hold, and, as you exhale, become more relaxed.

Eye Closure

You will then hear the suggestion that your eyelids can feel heavy, and as you take another deep breath of air you will allow your eyelids to close.

Achieving Hypnotic Relaxation

After your eyes are closed, you will receive additional suggestions for relaxation. These will include noticing a "wave of relaxation" that spreads from the top of your head to the bottom of your feet. I will give you suggestions to become more relaxed, physically, mentally, and emotionally.

As you become more absorbed in your own experience you may notice some changes in feelings and sensations. You may be aware that you are in a very deeply relaxed state, or that you are experiencing a feeling of heaviness, a floating feeling, or coolness.

Mental Imagery

I will then provide you with suggestions to experience mental imagery for coolness. I will give you an indication to drift into your own, individualized mental imagery for relaxation and coolness. You may experience a cool breeze, cool mountain air, a cool mist, or snow around you. For Emily, it involved a memory of walking down to a lake in Michigan on an evening where she could feel a cool breeze. Your mental imagery is your own, and there are no limits because you are now learning what works best for you!

Posthypnotic Suggestions

Next will be suggestions for additional changes to occur in the weeks ahead. Suggestions will be given for better sleep, feeling less stress, and reducing frequency and severity of hot flashes.

Alerting

I'll give you suggestions for returning to conscious alertness. I'll present some numbers with the suggestion that each number can serve as a cue to return to conscious alertness. You may return to alertness or you may drift off into sleep. It is your choice and in your control.

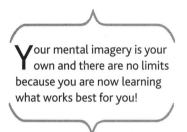

Your mental imagery is your own and there are no limits because you are now learning what works best for you!

As you will be encouraged to do weekly, it is important to review the "Ten Steps to Successful Practice of Hypnotic Relaxation for Hot Flashes," as these will keep you on track and aware of your practices.

**Ten Steps to Successful Practice of
Hypnotic Relaxation for Hot Flashes**

1. Find a quiet place to practice.
2. Make arrangements to avoid interruptions.
3. Do not engage in any other activity during your practice time.
4. Rate your level of relaxation before practice and after.
5. Focus your attention on the audio recording.
6. Adopt an attitude of "letting go" and calmness.
7. Notice relaxation.
8. Notice mental images and feelings of coolness.
9. Have an awareness of when and how to practice that works best for you.
10. Maintain your "Hot Flash Daily Diary."

LET'S BEGIN

Now go ahead and find a comfortable place to lie down or sit to listen to the audio file entitled, *Individualizing Hypnotic Relaxation for Hot Flashes.*

Before beginning your hypnotic relaxation session please rate your level of relaxation.

0------1------2------3------4------5------6------7------8------9------10

No relaxation at all   As relaxed as I possibly could be

Once you have completed your session today, you should complete your postsession rating and notes.

POSTSESSION

Upon completion of your hypnotic relaxation session please rate your level of relaxation again.

0------1------2------3------4------5------6------7------8------9------10

No relaxation at all   As relaxed as I possibly could be

Now jot down a few notes regarding your experience. Please reflect on and make notes regarding the following questions.

What were you most aware of when you opened your eyes after listening to the audio recording?

_____

_____

Which part of the audio recording did you like the best?

_____

_____

Were there some suggestions that seemed to help you relax the most?

_____

_____

What were your personal and individualized mental images for coolness and relaxation (mountains, lake, another place where you visualized coolness)?

_____

_____

Did you notice any other images or memories that helped you to become relaxed and find coolness?

_____

_____

IN THE WEEK AHEAD

Continue to Practice Daily, One or More Times a Day

Use the recording that accompanies this chapter, *Individualizing Hypnotic Relaxation for Hot Flashes*, at least one time each day in the upcoming week. If you are able to practice additional times per day, you may wish to use either of the recordings from Week 1, *Hypnotic Relaxation Therapy for Hot Flashes-Mountain Imagery* or *Hypnotic Relaxation Therapy for Hot Flashes-Lake Imagery.*

Continue to Maintain Your Hot Flash Daily Diary

It is generally expected that you will see a decrease of as much as 40% after the second full week of daily practice of hypnotic relaxation therapy.

At the end of this chapter you will find a blank Hot Flash Daily Diary for Week 2

Continue to Track Your Triggers

Note any situations where you tend to have hot flashes. This information can help guide your practice. Please continue to write down any triggers that you notice. This can give you important information about things that may contribute to your hot flashes that you may want to change as your progress through the program. Common triggers are stress, certain foods, habits, or situations.

At the end of this chapter you will find a blank Hot Flash Triggers form.

Complete a Relaxation Practice Checklist

At the end of this chapter you will find a blank Hypnotic Relaxation Practice Checklist for Week 2. It is important to continue to record your practice so you can see how frequently you are using hypnotic relaxation and track your progress in achieving relaxation during each daily session.

Look forward to a successful week of practice!

Go to the appendix or www.demoshealth.com/store/
elkins-relief-from-hot-flashes-supplements to access
additional blank copies of the:
Hot Flash Daily Diary
Hot Flash Triggers form
Hypnotic Relaxation Practice Checklist

Week 2
HOT FLASH DAILY DIARY

| Date | Make a mark for each hot flash to indicate mild, moderate, severe, or very severe | | | | Total # of Hot Flashes Today | NOTES (Use this space to record possible triggers or other information relating to trends you may notice about your hot flashes) |
	MILD	MODE-RATE	SEVERE	VERY SEVERE		
MON						
TUES						
WEDS						
THURS						
FRI						
SAT						
SUN						
TOTALS						

Severity Descriptors

Mild	Lasts <5 minutes; uncomfortable warmth; mild discomfort; no need for action
Moderate	Up to 15 minutes; warm, clammy skin; increased heart rate; some sweating; agitated; embarrassed; use fan, remove clothes, etc.
Severe	Up to 20 minutes; very hot; increased heart rate; unusual sensation over skin; sweating; anxiety; embarrassment; activity interruption
Very severe	Up to 45 minutes; extreme heat; rolling perspiration; increased heart rate; nausea; extreme distress; difficulty functioning; need to take cold shower or hold ice on skin

WEEK 2 HOT FLASH TRIGGERS

POTENTIAL TRIGGER	ACTIVITY

Week 2
HYPNOTIC RELAXATION
PRACTICE CHECKLIST

DATE: _____

Week #: ○ 1 ○ 2 ○ 3 ○ 4 ○ 5

1. *During the past week,* how often have you practiced hypnotic relaxation with the audio recording?

Daily (seven times per week) or more	☐
Three to six times per week	☐
One to two times per week	☐
None	☐

2. Please rate your average relaxation before hypnotic relaxation (Presession average):

    0   1   2   3   4   5   6   7   8   9   10

No   Extremely

relaxation   relaxed

3. Please rate your average relaxation after hypnotic relaxation (Postsession average):

    0   1   2   3   4   5   6   7   8   9   10

No   Extremely

relaxation   relaxed

Chapter 14

Week 3: Learning Self-Hypnosis for Hot Flashes

The audio file entitled *Learning Self-Hypnosis* accompanies this chapter*

This week you will learn how to add a brief self-hypnosis practice to your daily practice with the audio recordings. It will be important that you use *both* the audio recordings and self-hypnosis to enhance your reduction of hot flashes. First, let's review your progress.

REVIEW YOUR WEEK 2 HOT FLASH DAILY DIARY AND CALCULATE YOUR HOT FLASH SCORE

Review your Hot Flash Daily Diary for Week 2 of practice to see how you are doing at this point in the program. Also, you will want to calculate your hot flash score for this past week. Using the severity point values, take a moment now to calculate your Week 2 hot flash score.

- One point for a **mild** hot flash
- Two points for a **moderate** hot flash

---

* To access these files, visit www.demoshealth.com/store/elkins-relief-from-hot-flashes-supplements

- Three points for a **severe** hot flash
- Four points for a **very severe** hot flash

Add up the number of hot flashes that you had for each category of severity rating.

Mild: Number of mild hot flashes multiplied times 1 = _____

Moderate: Number of moderate hot flashes multiplied times 2 = _____

Severe: Number of severe hot flashes multiplied times 3 = _____

Very severe: Number of very severe hot flashes multiplied times 4 = _____

Add up the total to get your total hot flash score for the week = _____

Now that you have your hot flash score for the week, you can determine the percentage of reduction of your hot flashes in comparison to your baseline hot flash score.

CALCULATE THE PERCENTAGE REDUCTION IN YOUR HOT FLASH SCORE IN COMPARION TO YOUR BASELINE

You will be able to see how much your hot flashes are decreasing by determining the percentage of decease in your hot flash score in comparison to your baseline score. As previously noted, this can be done by a calculation of the percentage of change in hot flash scores in comparison to your baseline hot flash score. To calculate this percentage, follow the steps below.

Subtract the current week's hot flash score from your baseline hot flash score.

_____ Baseline hot flash score

− _____ Weekly hot flash score

= _____ Difference

Divide the difference by the baseline hot flash score

_____ Difference

/ _____ Baseline hot flash score

= _____ Quotient

Multiply the quotient times 100 to determine the percentage of decrease.

_____ Quotient

× _____ 100

= _____ %

Here are three specific things to look for:

- Did the number of hot flashes decrease from the previous week?
- Is there a shift from severe/very severe toward mild/moderate in the severity rating of hot flashes?
- How does your hot flash score for this week compare to your baseline hot flash score?

If your hot flash score decreased between 35% and 45%, you are perfectly on course at this stage of your program! If you do not see that range of decrease, then you will need to carefully review your Hypnotic Relaxation Practice Checklist to see what modifications may need to be made. As an example, we can take a look at Emily's hot flash score and her percentage reduction for the week.

HOW DID EMILY DO?

Hot Flash Score

As you review Emily's Week 2 Hot Flash Daily Diary, you can see that her hot flashes are less frequent and the severity of her hot flashes has shown a slight shift to the left.

Mild: 4 hot flashes   × 1 =   1

Moderate: 13 hot flashes × 2 = 26

Severe: 14 hot flashes × 3 = 42

Very Severe: 4 hot flashes   × 4 = 16

                              88 = Emily's Week 2 Hot Flash Score

Reduction Percentage

Step 1: Subtract the current week's hot flash score from the baseline hot flash score.

　　146   Emily's baseline hot flash score

　　−88   Emily's Week 2 hot flash score

　　　58   Difference

Step 2: Divide the difference by the baseline hot flash score

　　58/146 = .40

Step 3: Multiply the quotient times 100 to determine the percentage of decrease.

　　.40 × 100 = 40%

Emily has experienced a 40% reduction in her hot flash score after two weeks of following the *Relief from Hot Flashes* program.

Emily's Week 2
HOT FLASH DAILY DIARY

Date	Make a mark for each hot flash to indicate mild, moderate, severe, or very severe				Total # of Hot Flashes Today	NOTES (Use this space to record possible triggers or other information relating to trends you may notice about your hot flashes)
	MILD	**MODE-RATE**	**SEVERE**	**VERY SEVERE**		
MON 8/6/xx	I	III	II	I	7	Stress at work, then shopping 1x with night sweats
TUES 8/7/xx		II	III	I	6	Stress; worked in garden for 3 hours – 2 severe! Woke 2x with night sweats
WEDS 8/8/xx	II	II	II		6	Stress at work— deadlines Company for dinner
THURS 8/9/xx		II	I	I	4	A good day! Only milds!!!
FRI 8/10/xx	I	II	II		5	Ate at Favorite Mexican restaurant; spicy food and margarita; one at night
SAT 8/11/xx		I	II	I	4	Mostly mild; none at night
SUN 8/12/xx		I	II		3	Another good day
TOTALS	4	13	14	4	35	

Severity Descriptors

Mild	Lasts <5 minutes; uncomfortable warmth; mild discomfort; no need for action
Moderate	Up to 15 minutes; warm, clammy skin; increased heart rate; some sweating; agitated; embarrassed; use fan, remove clothes, etc.
Severe	Up to 20 minutes; very hot; increased heart rate; unusual sensation over skin; sweating; anxiety; embarrassment; activity interruption
Very severe	Up to 45 minutes; extreme heat; rolling perspiration; increased heart rate; nausea; extreme distress; difficulty functioning; need to take cold shower or hold ice on skin

REVIEW YOUR HYPNOTIC RELAXATION PRACTICE CHECKLIST AND TRIGGERS

OK, next, take a moment to look over your Hypnotic Relaxation Practice Checklist for the past week. Review how many times you were able to practice. As you review the checklist, reflect on the exact time you practiced each day and if you missed any days. Does your average rating of relaxation show that you became more relaxed after a practice session, and are you reducing hot flashes? If not, a few ideas are listed below.

- Be sure you are practicing hypnotic relaxation often enough.
- If you lie down and fall asleep each time you practice, schedule some times during the day when you are alert and sitting up.
- Don't try too hard. Remember, hypnotic relaxation is a process of "letting go." Learning to "let go" of worries can get easier with daily practice of hypnotic relaxation therapy.
- Find an individual mental image of relaxation, safety, coolness, and positive feelings that you can most easily identify with. This should be from personal experience but can come from childhood or any other time.
- Review the "Ten Steps to Successful Practice of Hypnotic Relaxation for Hot Flashes" to be sure you are using all the steps!

Also, review your form for recording any triggers. At this point you may or may not have identified any new triggers. However, being aware of potential triggers can give you more control over hot flashes as you note the things you can or have changed for your own benefit.

EMILY'S WEEK 2 HYPNOTIC RELAXATION PRACTICE CHECKLIST

Emily continued to practice hypnotic relaxation with the audio recordings at least once per day. You can review her Hypnotic Relaxation Practice Checklist and see that her practice was consistent and that she is becoming more relaxed and less stressed. Her hot flashes are decreasing as expected. She has not identified any new triggers, but feels she is making good progress.

Emily's Week 2
HYPNOTIC RELAXATION
PRACTICE CHECKLIST

DATE: 8/12/xx

Week #:   ○ 1   ⊗ 2   ○ 3   ○ 4   ○ 5

1. *During the past week,* how often have you practiced hypnotic relaxation with the audio recording?

      Daily (seven times per week) or more   ☒

      Three to six times per week   ☐

      One to two times per week   ☐

      None   ☐

2. Please rate your average relaxation before hypnotic relaxation (Presession average):

      0   1   2   3   ④   5   6   7   8   9   10
      No   Extremely
      relaxation   relaxed

3. Please rate your average relaxation after hypnotic relaxation (Postsession average):

      0   1   2   3   4   5   6   7   ⑧   9   10
      No   Extremely
      relaxation   relaxed

STARTING WEEK 3

In the third week ahead you will learn to add the use of self-hypnosis to your practice of hypnotic relaxation for reducing hot flashes. If you have not made the progress you desire, adding self-hypnosis practice can greatly increase your progress and is an important part of your overall success in reducing hot flashes and keeping them under control.

Let me begin by explaining what I mean by "self-hypnosis." In the start of this program, and up until now, all of your practice of hypnotic relaxation has been with the use of audio recordings. This daily practice with the audio recordings is something that you should continue to do. However, you can also benefit from learning how to achieve a hypnotic state and experience mental imagery for relaxation and coolness on your own, without using the recordings. This is self-hypnosis—a method of achieving hypnotic relaxation through your own practice.

> The advantage of adding self-hypnosis is that you can practice it at any place and time that is appropriate for you...

The advantage of adding self-hypnosis is that you can practice it at any place and time that is appropriate for you, even if you do not have access to an audio recording. Also, the method of self-hypnosis that I will show you can be very brief, lasting as little as four or five minutes. Thus, you may practice self-hypnosis between four and ten times a day. You can decide on how frequently and where you need to practice to bring your hot flashes down even further.

The methods of self-hypnosis are easy to learn and can be learned with practice.

WHAT TO EXPECT ON THE AUDIO RECORDING

Please look over the self-hypnosis instructions below because you will reference them as you practice. As you listen to the audio recording it will guide you through four self-hypnosis practice sessions. The first will be completely guided. In the second practice session you will be given prompts for the instructions on the facing page.

In the third practice session you will be given very minimal prompts, and in the fourth practice session you will not be given any prompts. In this way you will learn self-hypnosis and have a tool so that you can do hypnotic relaxation even when you do not have access to audio recordings or have limited time to practice.

The audio recording for *Learning Self-Hypnosis* that you will be using will direct you to look at these instructions at various times.

1. Roll eyes upward and focus on a spot.
2. Take a deep breath of air, and as you exhale, allow your eyelids to close.
3. Now, focus on your breathing. With each breath of air you breathe out, think the word "relax" and allow your body to become more relaxed. The mind and the body are working together for a common purpose ... to create feelings of relaxation and comfort.
4. Now, notice a wave of relaxation that spreads from the top of your head down to the bottom of your feet. Across your forehead, neck, shoulders, arms, back, chest and stomach, legs and feet. Every muscle and every fiber of your body ... more and more completely relaxed.
5. Now, with one part of your mind, go to another place. A place where you are safe and feel secure ... calm, and at ease. Going to that place now ... where you find coolness and comfort. That place may be in the mountains with snow all around ... in front of an air conditioner ... standing in a cool shower ... or another place where you find feelings of safety and deep relaxation ... coolness and comfort.
6. Now, as you are there ... Deepen this hypnotic relaxation ... going even deeper relaxed. Not only deeply relaxed *physically,* but also *emotionally relaxed* ... calm ... more at peace, and more at ease. And *mentally calm and relaxed* ... relaxed within your thoughts and feelings and physically deeply relaxed and comfortable.
7. And as you are there ... in that pleasant place ... so relaxed that you may notice a floating feeling, a tingly sensation ... or a numbness ... less aware of your body... nothing bothers and nothing disturbs.
8. And allowing this comfort and coolness to continue ... in some way remaining more relaxed and at ease ... feeling more in

control of your feelings and allowing a feeling of well-being to continue.

9. Now, go even a little deeper relaxed... deepen the hypnotic relaxation even more now. Head, neck, arms, back, chest and stomach, legs and feet ... completely relaxed ... and so cool and comfortable. Releasing every worry and every tension now.

10. And now ... gently and easily ... returning to conscious alertness ... in your own time and your own pace ... in a way that pleases you.

Learning self-hypnosis takes practice. With time, you will find that you are able to achieve a very relaxed state without using the hypnotic relaxation recordings. However, as you are learning this skill, it is very important that you continue to use both methods of daily practice. This is a learned skill that enhances your natural ability to relax your mind and body, and as with any skill, it takes practice.

**Ten Steps to Successful Practice of
Hypnotic Relaxation for Hot Flashes**

1. Find a quiet place to practice.
2. Make arrangements to avoid interruptions.
3. Do not engage in any other activity during your practice time.
4. Rate your level of relaxation before practice and after.
5. Focus your attention on the audio recording.
6. Adopt an attitude of "letting go" and calmness.
7. Notice relaxation.
8. Notice mental images and feelings of coolness.
9. Have an awareness of when and how to practice that works best for you.
10. Maintain your Hot Flash Daily Diary.

LET'S BEGIN

Sit in a comfortable position and in a place where you will not be disturbed. Rate your level of relaxation.

0------1------2------3------4------5------6------7------8------9------10

No relaxation at all   As relaxed as I possibly could be

Now, play the audio recording entitled, *Learning Self-Hypnosis*. After you listen to the recording you should complete the postsession ratings.

POSTSESSION

After your hypnotic relaxation session, please rate your level of relaxation again.

0------1------2------3------4------5------6------7------8------9------10

No relaxation at all   As relaxed as I possibly could be

Also, after you listen to the audio recording, jot down a few notes regarding your experience today. Please reflect on and make a few notes regarding the following questions.

What were you most aware of when you opened your eyes after listening to the audio recording?

_____

_____

Which part of the audio recording did you like the best?

_____

_____

Were there some suggestions that seemed to help you relax the most?

_____

_____

Did you experience some aspects of the mental images (mountains, lake, coolness) that were suggested?

_____

_____

Did you notice any other images or memories that helped you to become relaxed and find coolness?

_____

_____

IN THE WEEK AHEAD

Continue to Practice Daily, One or More Times a Day

Each day, have at least one hypnotic relaxation practice session. In the week ahead you should continue to use one of the audio files of your choice: *Individualizing Hypnotic Relaxation for Hot Flashes, Hypnotic Relaxation Therapy for Hot Flashes-Mountain Imagery,* or *Hypnotic Relaxation Therapy for Hot Flashes-Lake Imagery.* Whichever one you prefer to use will be the best one for your daily practice. In addition, you should begin daily self-hypnosis.

Add Self-Hypnosis to the 30-Minute Audio Recording Sessions

Some guidelines for your practice of daily self-hypnosis are:
- Practice self-hypnosis several times a day.
- Self-hypnosis practice may last about four to five minutes at a time.
- Self-hypnosis practice can be between four and ten times a day.
- The frequency of self-hypnosis practice should be based on what you need to progress further in the reduction of your hot flashes.
- You may refer to the written script in this chapter to guide your practice.

Continue to Maintain Your Hot Flash Daily Diary

It is generally expected that you will see a decrease of as much as 50% after the third full week of daily practice of hypnotic relaxation therapy. This is very, very important so you can track your progress!

At the end of this chapter you will find a blank Hot Flash Daily Diary for Week 3

Continue to Track Your Triggers

Note any situations where you tend to have hot flashes. This information can help guide your practice. Especially, write down any new triggers you may notice. For example, if there have been any significant changes in your life over the past few weeks, they may have caused stress that could be a trigger. If you have not noticed any new triggers or changes, then that is fine and you may already be aware of any potential triggers.

At the end of this chapter you will find a blank Hot Flash Triggers form.

Complete a Relaxation Practice Checklist

At the end of this chapter you will find a blank Hypnotic Relaxation Practice Checklist for Week 3. Please continue to record how frequently you have been practicing hypnotic relaxation using the audio recordings. Also, note how frequently you have practiced self-hypnosis without the audio recordings. Research has shown that the frequency of practice is very important, and sufficient frequency is necessary for success. Especially note if you have encountered any barriers to achieving daily practice.

Best wishes for a great week ahead!

Go to the appendix or www.demoshealth.com/store/elkins-relief-from-hot-flashes-supplements to access additional blank copies of the:
Hot Flash Daily Diary
Hot Flash Triggers form
Hypnotic Relaxation Practice Checklist

Week 3
HOT FLASH DAILY DIARY

Date	Make a mark for each hot flash to indicate mild, moderate, severe, or very severe				Total # of Hot Flashes Today	NOTES (Use this space to record possible triggers or other information relating to trends you may notice about your hot flashes)
	MILD	MODE-RATE	SEVERE	VERY SEVERE		
MON / /	___	___	___	___		
TUES / /	___	___	___	___		
WEDS / /	___	___	___	___		
THURS / /	___	___	___	___		
FRI / /	___	___	___	___		
SAT / /	___	___	___	___		
SUN / /	___	___	___	___		
TOTALS						

Severity Descriptors

Mild	Lasts <5 minutes; uncomfortable warmth; mild discomfort; no need for action
Moderate	Up to 15 minutes; warm, clammy skin; increased heart rate; some sweating; agitated; embarrassed; use fan, remove clothes, etc.
Severe	Up to 20 minutes; very hot; increased heart rate; unusual sensation over skin; sweating; anxiety; embarrassment; activity interruption
Very severe	Up to 45 minutes; extreme heat; rolling perspiration; increased heart rate; nausea; extreme distress; difficulty functioning; need to take cold shower or hold ice on skin

WEEK 3 HOT FLASH TRIGGERS

POTENTIAL TRIGGER	ACTIVITY

Week 3
HYPNOTIC RELAXATION
PRACTICE CHECKLIST

DATE: _____

Week #:   ○ 1   ○ 2   ○ 3   ○ 4   ○ 5

1. *During the past week,* how often have you practiced hypnotic relaxation with the audio recording?

    Daily (seven times per week) or more   ☐

    Three to six times per week   ☐

    One to two times per week   ☐

    None   ☐

2. Please rate your average relaxation before hypnotic relaxation (Presession average):

    0   1   2   3   4   5   6   7   8   9   10

    No   Extremely
    relaxation   relaxed

3. Please rate your average relaxation after hypnotic relaxation (Postsession average):

    0   1   2   3   4   5   6   7   8   9   10

    No   Extremely
    relaxation   relaxed

Chapter 15

Week 4: Knowing Your Body and Controlling Your Hot Flashes

The audio file entitled *Hypnotic Relaxation for Hot Flashes: Awareness and Control* accompanies this chapter.[*]

Congratulations on completing Week 3! To this point you have learned the method of hypnotic relaxation, identified some individual mental imagery, and begun practice of a brief self-hypnosis technique. The goal during Week 4 is to continue your progress by using hypnotic relaxation to increase awareness of your body. Having a greater awareness of your body and knowing how you experience relaxation can help you achieve more control over hot flashes.

First, let's review your progress.

REVIEW YOUR WEEK 3 HOT FLASH DAILY DIARY AND CALCULATE YOUR HOT FLASH SCORE

Please take a look at your Week 3 Hot Flash Daily Diary and calculate your hot flash score.

---

[*] To access these files, visit www.demoshealth.com/store/elkins-relief-from-hot-flashes-supplements

Using the severity point values, take a moment now to calculate your Week 3 hot flash score.

- one point for a **mild** hot flash
- two points for a **moderate** hot flash
- three points for a **severe** hot flash
- four points for a **very severe** hot flash

Add up the number of hot flashes that you had for each category of severity rating.

Mild: Number of mild hot flashes multiplied times 1 = _____

Moderate: Number of moderate hot flashes multiplied times 2 = _____

Severe: Number of severe hot flashes multiplied times 3 = _____

Very severe: Number of very severe hot flashes multiplied times 4 = _____

Add up the total to get your total hot flash score for the week = _____

Now, calculate your percentage of reduction of hot flash score for this past week. The formula for calculating this percentage is provided below.

CALCULATE THE PERCENTAGE REDUCTION IN YOUR HOT FLASH SCORE IN COMPARION TO YOUR BASELINE

To calculate the percentage of reduction in your hot flash score after three weeks of hypnotic relaxation therapy practice, follow the steps below.

Subtract the current week's hot flash score from your baseline hot flash score.

_____ Baseline hot flash score

− _____ Weekly hot flash score

= _____ Difference

Divide the difference by the baseline hot flash score

_____ Difference

/ _____ Baseline hot flash score

= _____ Quotient

Multiply the quotient times 100 to determine the percentage of decrease.

_____ Quotient

× _____ 100

= _____ %

Here are three specific things to look for:

- Did the number of hot flashes decrease from the previous week?
- Is there a shift from severe/very severe toward mild/moderate in the severity rating of hot flashes?
- How does your hot flash score for this week compare to your baseline hot flash score?

If your hot flashes decreased by 50% to 60%, you are perfectly on course with your program at this stage of progress!

HOW DID EMILY DO?

As you look at Emily's Hot Flash Daily Diary for the past week (p. 167), you can see that both the frequency and severity of hot flashes decreased as she began to use self-hypnosis as well as continuing to use the audio file recordings. Her preference was to use the audio file *Hypnotic Relaxation for Hot Flashes-Lake Imagery,* and she was using this each evening as well as practicing self-hypnosis several times during the day.

Hot Flash Score

As you review Emily's Week 3 Hot Flash Daily Diary, you can see that her hot flashes are less frequent and the severity of her hot flashes continues its trend of a slight shift to the left.

Mild: 2 hot flashes × 1 = 2
Moderate: 14 hot flashes × 2 = 28
Severe: 10 hot flashes × 3 = 30
Very severe: 3 hot flashes × 4 = 12
                              72 = Emily's Week 3 Hot Flash
                                   Score

Reduction Percentage

Step 1: Subtract the current week's hot flash score from the baseline hot flash score.

   146   Emily's baseline hot flash score

   − 72   Emily's Week 3 hot flash score

   74   Difference

Step 2: Divide the difference by the baseline hot flash score

   58/146 = 0.51

Step 3: Multiply the quotient times 100 to determine the percentage of decrease.

   0.51 × 100 = 51%

Emily has experienced a 51% reduction in her hot flash score after three weeks of following the Hypnotic Relaxation Therapy program. While this reduction is within the range of progress (50%–60%), Emily felt that she was "slipping" and wanted to make some changes. Though we were not terribly concerned, Emily and I discussed this and ways that she could adjust her practices in order to maximize her progress. It was her decision to incorporate the individualized recording into her practices in addition to what she was already doing, for at least four days in the upcoming week. Emily is committed and has done well, and I hope you did too!

Emily's Week 3
HOT FLASH DAILY DIARY

Date	Make a mark for each hot flash to indicate mild, moderate, severe, or very severe				Total # of Hot Flashes Today	NOTES (Use this space to record possible triggers or other information relating to trends you may notice about your hot flashes)
	MILD	**MODE-RATE**	**SEVERE**	**VERY SEVERE**		
MON 8/13/xx		III	I	I	5	Only 1 night sweat Stress-shopping
TUES 8/14/xx		II	II		4	Kids and grandkids over for dinner—hectic
WEDS 8/15/xx		II	II		4	No triggers really
THURS 8/16/xx	I	III	I		5	Two glasses of wine with dinner
FRI 8/17/xx	I	I	I	I	4	Stress—exciting ball game
SAT 8/18/xx		I	II	I	4	Worked in the garden
SUN 8/19/xx		II	I		3	Good day!
TOTALS	2	14	10	3	29	

Severity Descriptors

Mild	Lasts <5 minutes; uncomfortable warmth; mild discomfort; no need for action
Moderate	Up to 15 minutes; warm, clammy skin; increased heart rate; some sweating; agitated; embarrassed; use fan, remove clothes, etc.
Severe	Up to 20 minutes; very hot; increased heart rate; unusual sensation over skin; sweating; anxiety; embarrassment; activity interruption
Very severe	Up to 45 minutes; extreme heat; rolling perspiration; increased heart rate; nausea; extreme distress; difficulty functioning; need to take cold shower or hold ice on skin

REVIEW YOUR HYPNOTIC RELAXATION PRACTICE CHECKLIST AND ANY TRIGGERS

Please also take a look at your Hypnotic Relaxation Practice Checklist. Notice how many times you practiced hypnotic relaxation using an audio recording. Did you practice at least once a day? Notice when and where you practiced that seemed most effective for you.

Also, notice how many times you practiced self-hypnosis without an audio recording. Did you practice at least four times a day? Did you practice more than four times a day? Please take a moment to reflect on when and where you used the self-hypnosis technique that seemed most effective and helpful for you.

Did you notice any new triggers for hot flashes? How are you dealing with these triggers? Have you made any changes in diet, stress, or activities that have helped you to reduce hot flashes? Reviewing any triggers can help you know the things that you can do to gain greater control of hot flashes in addition to daily practice of hypnotic relaxation.

EMILY'S WEEK 3 HYPNOTIC RELAXATION PRACTICE CHECKLIST

A review of Emily's practice of hypnotic relaxation shows that during the third week of the program she continued to practice hypnotic relaxation therapy at least daily. She reported to me that she was using the audio recordings primarily at night and this was likely to help her sleep better. Remember that one of the benefits of regular hypnotic relaxation therapy practice is improved sleep. Her Hypnotic Relaxation Practice Checklist for Week 3 is provided for your review. You can see that she was achieving quite a bit of relaxation with her practice! In addition, she indicated to me that she was practicing self-hypnosis about four times per day. She found that she could most easily use self-hypnosis at work during her morning break and for about five minutes during her lunch break. She stated that she also practiced a brief self-hypnosis session right before potentially stressful situations such as before a class that she was teaching.

Emily's Week 3
HYPNOTIC RELAXATION
PRACTICE CHECKLIST

DATE: 8/19/xx

Week #: ○ 1   ○ 2   ⊗ 3   ○ 4   ○ 5

1. *During the past week,* how often have you practiced hypnotic relaxation with the audio recording?

     Daily (seven times per week) or more   ☐

     Three to six times per week   ☐

     One to two times per week   ☒

     None   ☐

2. Please rate your average relaxation before hypnotic relaxation (presession average):

     0   1   2   3   4   5   (6)   7   8   9   10

     No   Extremely
     relaxation   relaxed

3. Please rate your average relaxation after hypnotic relaxation (postsession average):

     0   1   2   3   4   5   6   7   8   (9)   10

     No   Extremely
     relaxation   relaxed

IMPROVING YOUR DAILY PRACTICE

Not everyone is the same and results will vary, but if your hot flash score isn't improving at a similar rate as Emily's, consider these factors and plan to make some changes to address them in the coming weeks:

- Daily practice:

    This is a vital aspect of this therapy program. Daily practice allows you to experience the relaxation process each day so that you become adept as learning to relax, visualize comfort and coolness, and become skilled at self-hypnosis.

- Practice location:

    It is important to practice your hypnotic relaxation in a location that is conducive to your physical comfort. You should be in a comfortable chair or lying on a bed. You may wish to elevate your feet. Your neck and lower back should be supported and not strained. The room should be quiet, with no interruptions.

- Practice time:

    When you practice your hypnotic relaxation is an individual choice based on your individual situational availability and preference. Many find that practicing at bedtime works well for them. However, others report they fall asleep and don't tend to see the reduction as quickly or fully as others. If you do like to practice at bedtime, that is fine; however, if you don't feel you are seeing the results you expect, try practicing at another time of day *in addition to* your bedtime practice.

- Perseverance:

    Whatever you do ... don't give up! Continue your practices; continue tracking your hot flashes on the Hot Flash Daily Dairy; and continue monitoring the things in your life that appear to trigger or have an association with your hot flashes.

STARTING WEEK 4

During week 4, you will continue to use the audio recordings of your preference, either *Hypnotic Relaxation for Hot Flashes-Mountain Imagery* or *Hypnotic Relaxation for Hot Flashes-Lake Imagery*, and practice self-hypnosis. In addition, you will have a session of hypnotic relaxation therapy using the audio recording entitled *Hypnotic Relaxation for Hot Flashes-Awareness and Control*; you may only listen to this particular recording once or twice, but you can repeat a session with this recording if you find it helpful.

It is likely that you are progressing well at this point and will make even more progress in the week ahead. If you are not progressing, it may be important for you to carefully make sure you are getting in enough practice of hypnotic relaxation therapy and using self-hypnosis effectively. Depending on your progress, it may be helpful to review the self-hypnosis instructions as well as the audio file for Week 4.

WHAT TO EXPECT ON THE AUDIO RECORDING

The audio recording *Hypnotic Relaxation for Hot Flashes: Awareness and Control* is similar to your previous practice and includes guidance to achieve relaxation as well as suggestions for increased control and positive mental imagery. It will proceed as follows:

Focus of Attention/Eye Closure

The practice session will begin by asking you to close your eyes, relax, and focus on your breathing.

Achieving Hypnotic Relaxation/Body Awareness

As you become more relaxed, I will suggest that you become more aware of your body and sensations.

As you become more deeply relaxed, I will ask you to notice any changes that occur in your breathing, sensations of coolness, and feelings of control.

Mental Imagery/Taking Control

I will then give you suggestions to experience mental imagery for coolness. As these suggestions are given, I will ask you to become more aware of your goals and taking control. Your personal goals may include sleeping better, reacting less to stress, decreasing hot flashes, or any other goal you might set for yourself.

Posthypnotic Suggestions

Suggestions will be given for greater body awareness and greater control in the weeks ahead. They will also be given for awareness of achieving your goals.

Alerting

Suggestions will then be given for returning to conscious alertness.

**Ten Steps to Successful Practice of
Hypnotic Relaxation for Hot Flashes**

1. Find a quiet place to practice.
2. Make arrangements to avoid interruptions.
3. Do not engage in any other activity during your practice time.
4. Rate your level of relaxation before practice and after.
5. Focus your attention on the audio recording.
6. Adopt an attitude of "letting go" and calmness.
7. Notice relaxation.
8. Notice mental images and feelings of coolness.
9. Have an awareness of when and how to practice that works best for you.
10. Maintain your Hot Flash Daily Diary.

LET'S BEGIN

As you prepare for your hypnotic relaxation session, find a comfortable place to sit or lie down where you will be free from distractions. Rate your level of relaxation before beginning.

0------1------2------3------4------5------6------7------8------9------10

No relaxation at all   As relaxed as I possibly could be

Begin your session, listen to the audio recording entitled *Hypnotic Relaxation for Hot Flashes: Awareness and Control,* and practice hypnotic relaxation. After you listen to the recording you should complete the postsession ratings.

POSTSESSION

Upon completion of your hypnotic relaxation session, please rate your level of relaxation again.

0------1------2------3------4------5------6------7------8------9------10

No relaxation at all   As relaxed as I possibly could be

After you listen to the audio recording, jot down a few notes regarding your experience today. Please reflect on and make a few notes regarding the following questions.

What sensations in your body were you most aware of during the hypnotic relaxation session today?

_____

_____

What changes did you notice as you became more deeply relaxed?

_____

_____

What were some of your personal goals that came into your awareness (better sleep, less stress, etc.)?

_____

_____

What were your personal and individualized mental images for coolness and relaxation and for achievement of your goals?

_____

_____

Did you notice any other images or memories today that helped you to become relaxed and find coolness?

_____

_____

IN THE WEEK AHEAD

Continue to Practice Daily, One or More times a Day

Use the audio file of your choice, either *Hypnotic Relaxation for Hot Flashes-Mountain Imagery, Hypnotic Relaxation for Hot Flashes-Lake Imagery,* or *Individualizing Hypnotic Relaxation for Hot Flashes.*
Continue your practice of self-hypnosis several times a day.

Continue to Maintain Your Hot Flash Daily Diary

It is generally expected that you will see a decrease of as much as 65% to 70% after the fourth full week of daily practice of hypnotic relaxation therapy.
At the end of this chapter you will find a blank Hot Flash Daily Diary for Week 4.

Continue to Track Your Triggers

Note any situations where you tend to have hot flashes. This information can help guide your practice. Continue to note any situations that serve as triggers or that are especially stressful for you. It is likely that these are either no longer as difficult or you may have already addressed the things that had been triggers in the past. Tracking your triggers will increase your awareness of them, and that awareness will help you to know situations you need to change or avoid, as well as when you should prectice self-hypnosis.

At the end of this chapter you will find a blank Hot Flash Triggers form.

Complete a Relaxation Practice Checklist

At the end of this chapter you will find a blank Hypnotic Relaxation Practice Checklist for Week 4. It is very important that you continue to record the frequency of your practice and how successful you are in achieving relaxation. This will help you know if you are practicing frequently enough and can help you build confidence in your ability to achieve a state of hypnotic relaxation.

Best wishes for another great week ahead!

Go to the appendix or www.demoshealth.com/store/elkins-relief-from-hot-flashes-supplements to access additional blank copies of the: Hot Flash Daily Diary Hot Flash Triggers form Hypnotic Relaxation Practice Checklist

Week 4
HOT FLASH DAILY DIARY

| Date | Make a mark for each hot flash to indicate mild, moderate, severe, or very severe | | | | Total # of Hot Flashes Today | NOTES (Use this space to record possible triggers or other information relating to trends you may notice about your hot flashes) |
	MILD	MODE-RATE	SEVERE	VERY SEVERE		
MON / /	___	___	___	___		
TUES / /	___	___	___	___		
WEDS / /	___	___	___	___		
THURS / /	___	___	___	___		
FRI / /	___	___	___	___		
SAT / /	___	___	___	___		
SUN / /	___	___	___	___		
TOTALS						

Severity Descriptors

Mild	Lasts <5 minutes; uncomfortable warmth; mild discomfort; no need for action
Moderate	Up to 15 minutes; warm, clammy skin; increased heart rate; some sweating; agitated; embarrassed; use fan, remove clothes, etc.
Severe	Up to 20 minutes; very hot; increased heart rate; unusual sensation over skin; sweating; anxiety; embarrassment; activity interruption
Very severe	Up to 45 minutes; extreme heat; rolling perspiration; increased heart rate; nausea; extreme distress; difficulty functioning; need to take cold shower or hold ice on skin

WEEK 4 HOT FLASH TRIGGERS

POTENTIAL TRIGGER	ACTIVITY

Week 4
HYPNOTIC RELAXATION
PRACTICE CHECKLIST

DATE: _____

Week #:   ○ 1   ○ 2   ○ 3   ○ 4   ○ 5

1. *During the past week,* how often have you practiced hypnotic relaxation with the audio recording?

    Daily (seven times per week) or more   ☐

    Three to six times per week   ☐

    One to two times per week   ☐

    None   ☐

2. Please rate your average relaxation before hypnotic relaxation (Presession average):

    0   1   2   3   4   5   6   7   8   9   10
    No   Extremely
    relaxation   relaxed

3. Please rate your average relaxation after hypnotic relaxation (Postsession average):

    0   1   2   3   4   5   6   7   8   9   10
    No   Extremely
    relaxation   relaxed

Chapter 16

Week 5: Setting Goals and Maintaining Your Progress

Over the past few weeks, you have been making hypnotic relaxation a part of your daily routine. This has included individualizing your practice, use of audio recordings, and frequent self-hypnosis. By recording your hot flashes with the Hot Flash Daily Diary you have been able to track your progress. Experience has shown that at this stage of the program most women begin to reduce their hot flashes by about 60% or more. Some women report greater reductions and some a bit less. The average is about 65% reduction compared to the start of the program.

Achieving even further reductions in hot flashes and maintaining your progress is largely dependent upon continued hypnotic relaxation therapy practice, so in this chapter we will review how you are doing and identify goals for maintaining your progress.

First, let's review your progress.

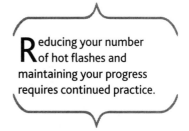

Reducing your number of hot flashes and maintaining your progress requires continued practice.

REVIEW YOUR WEEK 4 HOT FLASH DAILY DIARY AND CALCULATE YOUR HOT FLASH SCORE

Take a moment to look over your Hot Flash Daily Diary. You may notice a considerable shift in hot flashes toward the mild rating and a significant reduction in your hot flash score. Also, there are probably a lot *fewer* hot flashes than when you started. Now, calculate your hot flash score using the following formula.

- One point for a **mild** hot flash
- Two points for a **moderate** hot flash
- Three points for a **severe** hot flash
- Four points for a **very severe** hot flash

Add up the number of hot flashes that you had for each category of severity rating.

Mild: Number of mild hot flashes multiplied times 1 = _____

Moderate: Number of moderate hot flashes multiplied times 2 = _____

Severe: Number of severe hot flashes multiplied times 3 = _____

Very severe: Number of very severe hot flashes multiplied times 4 = _____

Add up the total to get your total hot flash score for the week = _____

How does it differ from your baseline score?

CALCULATE THE PERCENTAGE REDUCTION IN YOUR HOT FLASH SCORE IN COMPARISON TO YOUR BASELINE

By now you are probably getting to be familiar with the formula for calculating the percentage of change in your hot flash score in comparison to your baseline. To make it a bit easier to calculate I have provided the steps below.

Subtract the current week's hot flash score from your baseline hot flash score.

_____ Baseline hot flash score

– _____ Weekly hot flash score

= _____ Difference

Divide the difference by the baseline hot flash score

_____ Difference

/ _____ Baseline hot flash score

= _____ Quotient

Multiply the quotient times 100 to determine the percentage of decrease.

_____ Quotient

× _____ 100

= _____ %

Here are three specific things to look for:

- Did the number of hot flashes decrease from the previous week?
- Is there a shift from severe/very severe toward mild/moderate in the severity rating of hot flashes?
- How does your hot flash score for this week compare to your baseline hot flash score?

At this point you are likely to have a 55% to 70% reduction in hot flash scores. How does your reduction percentage compare to the average of about 65%? Let's now take a look at Emily's progress after four weeks of practice of hypnotic relaxation therapy and using self-hypnosis.

HOW DID EMILY DO?

Hot Flash Score

As you review Emily's Week 4 Hot Flash Daily Diary (p. 183), you can see that her hot flashes are less frequent and the severity of her hot flashes continues its trend of a slight shift to the left.

Mild: 5 hot flashes × 1 = 5
Moderate: 17 hot flashes × 2 = 34
Severe: 4 hot flashes × 3 = 12
Very severe: 0 hot flashes × 4 = 0

51 = Emily's Week 4 Hot
Flash Score

Reduction Percentage

Step 1: Subtract the current week's hot flash score from the baseline hot flash score.

146   Emily's baseline hot flash score

– 51   Emily's Week 4 hot flash score

95   Difference

Step 2: Divide the difference by the baseline hot flash score

$95/146 = .65$

Step 3: Multiply the quotient times 100 to determine the percentage of decrease.

$.65 × 100 = 65\%$

Emily's hot flash score for Week 4 was 51, a significant reduction from her baseline hot flash score of 146, which represents a 65% reduction!

How does your hot flash score reduction compare to Emily's? Are there any modifications in your practice of hypnotic relaxation therapy that might be helpful for you? For example, reflect on your frequency of practice with the audio recording and your use of self-hypnosis. Also, note if you have made any needed changes to deal with any particular hot flash triggers you have identified thus far.

Emily's Week 4
HOT FLASH DAILY DIARY

Date	Make a mark for each hot flash to indicate mild, moderate, severe, or very severe				Total # of Hot Flashes Today	NOTES (Use this space to record possible triggers or other information relating to trends you may notice about your hot flashes)
	MILD	MODE-RATE	SEVERE	VERY SEVERE		
MON 8/20/xx	I	II	I		4	Stress at work; used self-hypnosis
TUES 8/21/xx	I	II	I		4	Shopping; crowds!
WEDS 8/22/xx	I	III			4	
THURS 8/23/xx		II	I		3	Good day
FRI 8/24/xx	I	III			4	Almost not noticeable
SAT 8/25/xx	I	II	I		4	
SUN 8/26/xx		III			3	No night sweats all week!!!
TOTALS	5	17	4		26	

Severity Descriptors

Mild	Lasts <5 minutes; uncomfortable warmth; mild discomfort; no need for action
Moderate	Up to 15 minutes; warm, clammy skin; increased heart rate; some sweating; agitated; embarrassed; use fan, remove clothes, etc.
Severe	Up to 20 minutes; very hot; increased heart rate; unusual sensation over skin; sweating; anxiety; embarrassment; activity interruption
Very severe	Up to 45 minutes; extreme heat; rolling perspiration; increased heart rate; nausea; extreme distress; difficulty functioning; need to take cold shower or hold ice on skin

REVIEW YOUR HYPNOTIC RELAXATION PRACTICE CHECKLIST AND HOT FLASH TRIGGERS

Look over your Hypnotic Relaxation Practice Checklist for the past week. By reviewing your practice, you can see how frequently you are using the audio recordings as well as practicing self-hypnosis. Recording hot flashes and consistent practice of hypnotic relaxation are essential to your progress at this point. Also, review your hot flash triggers. At this point you may or may not have identified any new triggers (Emily did not), but it can still be helpful to notice if you still have any triggers for hot flashes, since it can indicate some things that you may need to avoid or change.

EMILY'S WEEK 4 HYPNOTIC RELAXATION PRACTICE CHECKLIST

Emily's Hypnotic Relaxation Practice Checklist is shown next. You can see that she has continued to practice with the audio recordings at least once per day. In fact, she indicated in session that she has slightly increased her practice to include day and night use of the recordings. Take a moment to compare your checklist to Emily's — it will give you a point of reference as you plan the week ahead!

Emily's Week 4
HYPNOTIC RELAXATION
PRACTICE CHECKLIST

DATE: 8/26/xx

Week #:   O 1   O 2   O 3   ⊗ 4   O 5

1. *During the past week,* how often have you practiced hypnotic relaxation with the audio recording?

    Daily (seven times per week) or more   ☒

    Three to six times per week   ☐

    One to two times per week   ☐

    None   ☐

2. Please rate your average relaxation before hypnotic relaxation (presession average):

    0   1   2   3   4   5   6   7   ⑧   9   10
    No   Extremely
    relaxation   relaxed

3. Please rate your average relaxation after hypnotic relaxation (postsession average):

    0   1   2   3   4   5   6   7   8   9   ⑩
    No   Extremely
    relaxation   relaxed

STARTING WEEK 5

Setting goals is an important part of hypnotic relaxation therapy. In the beginning of this program, your primary goal was to reduce hot flashes. It is likely that you have made progress toward that goal. There are also other benefits from hypnotic relaxation therapy. You may have noticed that you feel calmer in your everyday activities or that you are sleeping better. You probably have more awareness of your body, your emotions, and reactions to stress.

In Week 5, reflect on what you would like to accomplish in this final week of the program. Depending on your goals, you may adjust your practice of hypnotic relaxation therapy and use of the audio recordings. This week is different from the previous weeks in that the focus is more on *how you use hypnotic relaxation* rather than learning a new technique. A few examples of goals are:

- Further reduce hot flashes at night (night sweats).
- Go to sleep more quickly.
- Relax more deeply while using the audio recordings.
- Use self-hypnosis more often during the day.
- Use more mental images for coolness.
- Reduce feelings of stress and feel calmer.

What are your goals for this week? Please take a moment to write down your goals.

_____

_____

_____

_____

ADJUSTING YOUR PRACTICE OF HYPNOTIC RELAXATION THERAPY

After you have identified your goals for the coming week, you may need to adjust your practice of hypnotic relaxation therapy. This could include the time of day that you practice, selecting a different audio recording, or reviewing the methods of self-hypnosis. The decision is based on your personal goals and progress to date. If you are satisfied with your progress, there may not be much that you need to change! However, achieving your goals may mean some adjustments. Please take a moment to jot down any adjustments you think you might need to make to achieve your goals for this week. For example, you may have practiced throughout the past weeks only once a day, and some days you may not have been able to practice at all. If you feel that you have not reduced your hot flash score to a level consistent with the norm indicated in this book, I would recommend that you increase the number of practices and possibly consider practicing at a different time of day. One suggestion would be to wake up a half-hour earlier and practice first thing in the morning. Additionally, the self-hypnosis practice should not be underestimated. This practice may feel awkward in the beginning, but it plays a vital role in your success because it provides you with a tool that allows you control over your hot flashes, especially the severity of your hot flashes.

I plan to adjust my practice of hypnotic relaxation therapy with the following changes:

_____

_____

_____

_____

Ten Steps to Successful Practice of
Hypnotic Relaxation for Hot Flashes

1. Find a quiet place to practice.
2. Make arrangements to avoid interruptions.
3. Do not engage in any other activity during your practice time.
4. Rate your level of relaxation before practice and after.
5. Focus your attention on the audio recording.
6. Adopt an attitude of "letting go" and calmness.
7. Notice relaxation.
8. Notice mental images and feelings of coolness.
9. Have an awareness of when and how to practice that works best for you.
10. Maintain your Hot Flash Daily Diary.

LET'S BEGIN

There is no new audio recording for this week. You will use either *Hypnotic Relaxation for Hot Flashes-Mountain Imagery*, *Hypnotic Relaxation for Hot Flashes-Lake Imagery*, *Individualizing Hypnotic Relaxation for Hot Flashes*, or *Hypnotic Relaxation for Hot Flashes-Awareness and Control* for this practice session. Use the audio recording that you prefer. Reflect on your goals and any adjustments as you prepare to practice hypnotic relaxation.

Find a comfortable place to sit or lie down where you will not be disturbed for about 30 minutes. Rate your level of relaxation before beginning.

0------1------2------3------4------5------6------7------8------9------10

No relaxation at all   As relaxed as I possibly could be

Begin your session using the audio file of your preference. After you listen to the recording you should complete the postsession ratings.

POSTSESSION

Upon completion of your hypnotic relaxation session please rate your level of relaxation again.

0------1------2------3------4------5------6------7--------8------9------10

No relaxation at all   As relaxed as I possibly could be

Because this session is focused on your personal goals, jot down a few notes regarding your experience today. Note anything you noticed in regard to your feelings and any of the suggestions on the recording that you found especially helpful.

Notes:

_____

_____

_____

_____

IN THE WEEK AHEAD

Continue to Practice Daily, One or More Times a Day

If you are able to practice additional times per day, you may use a variation of the recordings you have received so far: *Hypnotic Relaxation for Hot Flashes-Mountain Imagery, Hypnotic Relaxation for Hot Flashes-Lake Imagery, Individualizing Hypnotic Relaxation for Hot Flashes,* or *Hypnotic Relaxation for Hot Flashes-Awareness and Control.*

Continue Self-Hypnosis Practice (in Addition to Using the Audio Files), One or More Times a Day

At this point you are probably becoming skilled in the use of self-hypnosis and have identified important times to use self-hypnosis to control your hot flashes. Continue your use of self-hypnosis as needed for reducing hot flashes even further this week.

Continue to Maintain Your Hot Flash Daily Diary

It is generally expected that you will see a decrease of as much as 65% to 70% or more after the fifth full week of daily practice of hypnotic relaxation therapy.

At the end of this chapter you will find a blank Hot Flash Daily Diary for Week 5

Continue to Track Your Triggers

Note any situations where you tend to have hot flashes. This information can help guide your practice. Note any new triggers and any things you have done to eliminate any triggers. Note any new stresses and how you are coping with stress.

At the end of this chapter you will find a blank Hot Flash Triggers form.

Complete a Relaxation Practice Checklist

At the end of this chapter you will find a blank Hypnotic Relaxation Practice Checklist for Week 5. It is important to continue to record the frequency of your practice of hypnotic relaxation and your response to it. This will give you very good information on how well you have been able to maintain daily practice, as well as an awareness of anything that can help you to continue your practice in the weeks ahead.

WEEK 6 AND BEYOND

At the end of this week, you will be ready to review your overall progress and achievement of all of your goals: reducing hot flashes, sleeping better, managing stress, and any other personal goals you have set for yourself. After you complete Week 5 of the program, read the next chapter.

Good luck for a great week ahead!

> Go to the appendix or www.demoshealth.com/store/elkins-relief-from-hot-flashes-supplements to access additional blank copies of the:
> Hot Flash Daily Diary
> Hot Flash Triggers form
> Hypnotic Relaxation Practice Checklist

Week 5
HOT FLASH DAILY DIARY

DATE	Make a mark for each hot flash to indicate mild, moderate, severe, or very severe				Total # of Hot Flashes Today	NOTES (Use this space to record possible triggers or other information relating to trends you may notice about your hot flashes)
	MILD	MODE-RATE	SEVERE	VERY SEVERE		
MON / /	____	____	____	____		
TUES / /	____	____	____	____		
WEDS / /	____	____	____	____		
THURS / /	____	____	____	____		
FRI / /	____	____	____	____		
SAT / /	____	____	____	____		
SUN / /	____	____	____	____		
TOTALS						

Severity Descriptors

Mild	Lasts <5 minutes; uncomfortable warmth; mild discomfort; no need for action
Moderate	Up to 15 minutes; warm, clammy skin; increased heart rate; some sweating; agitated; embarrassed; use fan, remove clothes, etc.
Severe	Up to 20 minutes; very hot; increased heart rate; unusual sensation over skin; sweating; anxiety; embarrassment; activity interruption
Very severe	Up to 45 minutes; extreme heat; rolling perspiration; increased heart rate; nausea; extreme distress; difficulty functioning; need to take cold shower or hold ice on skin

WEEK 5 HOT FLASH TRIGGERS

POTENTIAL TRIGGER	ACTIVITY

Week 5
HYPNOTIC RELAXATION
PRACTICE CHECKLIST

DATE: _____

Week #: ○ 1   ○ 2   ○ 3   ○ 4   ○ 5

1. *During the past week,* how often have you practiced hypnotic relaxation with the audio recording?

Daily (seven times per week) or more	☐
Three to six times per week	☐
One to two times per week	☐
None	☐

2. Please rate your average relaxation before hypnotic relaxation (Presession average):

0	1	2	3	4	5	6	7	8	9	10
No relaxation										Extremely relaxed

3. Please rate your average relaxation after hypnotic relaxation (Postsession average):

0	1	2	3	4	5	6	7	8	9	10
No relaxation										Extremely relaxed

Chapter 17

Assessing Your Progress

Y ou have watched weekly while your hot flashes have become less frequent and less severe as you have worked through this book and listened to your recordings. By completing the Hot Flash Daily Diary each week and comparing your weekly hot flash scores with your baseline diary you have been able to get a clear picture of your success.

Before beginning the program, you also completed a Sleep Rating Form and a Hot Flash Related Daily Interference Scale (HFRDIS) that captured a snapshot of where you were at that time with your sleep and emotional well-being. By completing these questionnaires again now that you have completed five weeks of practice with the hypnosis recordings, you will have a clear image of other changes that have been occurring in your life.

Just to make it interesting, don't look at your baseline measures until you have completed these assessments for the second time.

YOUR REDUCTION IN HOT FLASHES

You have completed the program of five weeks of listening to the hypnotic relaxation recordings, and now have a valuable tool that you will find extremely effective in managing your hot flashes and maintaining control of your life.

Let's review your Week 5 Hot Flash Daily Diary to see your overall progress.

REVIEW YOUR WEEK 5 HOT FLASH DAILY DIARY AND CALCULATE YOUR HOT FLASH SCORE

Take a moment to look over your weeks of Hot Flash Daily Diaries. There are probably now a lot fewer hot flashes than when you started, and the severity of the ones you are experiencing has likely shifted very much to mild/moderate. Now calculate your hot flash score using the following formula.

- one point for a **mild** hot flash
- two points for a **moderate** hot flash
- three points for a **severe** hot flash
- four points for a **very severe** hot flash

Add up the number of hot flashes that you had for each category of severity rating.

Mild: Number of mild hot flashes multiplied times 1 = _____

Moderate: Number of moderate hot flashes multiplied times 2 = _____

Severe: Number of severe hot flashes multiplied times 3 = _____

Very severe: Number of very severe hot flashes multiplied times 4 = _____

Add up the total to get your total hot flash score for the week = _____

How does your Week 5 hot flash score compare to your baseline hot flash score?

CALCULATE THE PERCENTAGE REDUCTION IN YOUR HOT FLASH SCORE IN COMPARION TO YOUR BASELINE

To calculate the percentage of reduction in your hot flash score after five weeks of hypnotic relaxation therapy practice, use the following steps.

Subtract the current week's hot flash score from your baseline hot flash score.

_____ Baseline hot flash score

−_____ Weekly hot flash score

=_____ Difference

Divide the difference by the baseline hot flash score.

_____ Difference

/_____ Baseline hot flash score

=_____ Quotient

Multiply the quotient times 100 to determine the percentage of decrease.

_____ Quotient

×_____ 100

=_____ %

Here are three specific things to look for:

- Did the number of hot flashes decrease from the baseline week?
- Is there a shift from severe/very severe toward mild/moderate in the severity rating of hot flashes?

How does your hot flash score for this week compare to your baseline hot flash score? The average reduction in hot flash scores at this point is about 70%. You may have achieved a lesser or greater reduction in hot flashes. *If your hot flashes have decreased by 50% or more, you have made excellent progress!*

ASSESSING THE CHANGE IN YOUR SLEEP

Sleep quality is important to your ability to function, and poor sleep quality can have negative effects on your physical health, work performance, and cognitive abilities. On the assessment you completed before you started the program, you can probably look back now and see that the majority of your responses fell to the left of the center, indicating that your sleep quality definitely needed improvement. Complete the Sleep Rating Form again now. I believe you will notice an improvement in your sleep quality from just five weeks ago.

Week 6
SLEEP RATING FORM

DATE: _____

During the past week, about how many hours did you sleep each night on average? ____

Circle the number that best represents your agreement with the following comments regarding your sleep *during the past week*.

	Not at all										Very much so
1. I was relaxed during my sleep.	0	1	2	3	4	5	6	7	8	9	10
2. I went to sleep quickly.	0	1	2	3	4	5	6	7	8	9	10
3. My sleep was good.	0	1	2	3	4	5	6	7	8	9	10
4. I awoke very few times during the night.	0	1	2	3	4	5	6	7	8	9	10
5. For my age, I felt like I got an adequate amount of sleep.	0	1	2	3	4	5	6	7	8	9	10
6. I was satisfied with my sleep.	0	1	2	3	4	5	6	7	8	9	10
7. My sleep met my expectations.	0	1	2	3	4	5	6	7	8	9	10
8. I was able to go to sleep without sleeping pills or drugs.	0	1	2	3	4	5	6	7	8	9	10
9. I stayed asleep most of the night.	0	1	2	3	4	5	6	7	8	9	10
10. I woke up feeling refreshed.	0	1	2	3	4	5	6	7	8	9	10

TOTAL SCORE: ____

("I slept well": 0 = not at all; 100 = very much so)

ASSESSING YOUR MOOD, RELATIONSHIPS, AND QUALITY OF LIFE RATINGS

In chapter 10, we discussed the Hot Flash Related Daily Interference Scale (HFRDIS) which provided a picture of how you viewed your quality of life (QOL) at that time. On this measure, you recorded a response to questions covering the following aspects of daily life:

- Work
- Social activities
- Leisure activities
- Sleep
- Mood
- Concentration
- Relations with others
- Sexuality
- Enjoyment of life

Now, complete the HFRDIS again. A copy is provided. I think you will find that there has been a positive change in many of these aspects of your daily life. Notice the areas where you have achieved improvement and how these have had a positive impact for you!

Go to the appendix or www.demoshealth.com/store/ elkins-relief-from-hot-flashes-supplements to access additional blank copies of the:
Sleep Rating Form
Hot Flash Related Daily Interference Scale (HFRDIS)

Week 6
HOT FLASH RELATED DAILY
INTERFERENCE SCALE (HFRDIS)

DATE: _____

Circle the number that best describes how much hot flashes have interfered with each aspect of your life *during the past week.*

	Not at all										Very much so
1. Work (work outside the home and house work)	0	1	2	3	4	5	6	7	8	9	10
2. Social activities (time spent with family, friends, etc.)	0	1	2	3	4	5	6	7	8	9	10
3. Leisure activities (time spent relaxing, doing hobbies, etc.)	0	1	2	3	4	5	6	7	8	9	10
4. Sleep	0	1	2	3	4	5	6	7	8	9	10
5. Mood	0	1	2	3	4	5	6	7	8	9	10
6. Concentration	0	1	2	3	4	5	6	7	8	9	10
7. Relations with others	0	1	2	3	4	5	6	7	8	9	10
8. Sexuality	0	1	2	3	4	5	6	7	8	9	10
9. Enjoyment of life	0	1	2	3	4	5	6	7	8	9	10
10. Overall quality of life	0	1	2	3	4	5	6	7	8	9	10

TOTAL SCORE: ___

("Hot flashes interfered with my life": 0 = not at all; 100 = very much so)

HOW DID EMILY DO AFTER FIVE WEEKS OF PRACTICE OF HYPNOTIC RELAXATION?

You can now take a look at Emily's progress by reviewing her Week 5 Hot Flash Daily Diary and the measures of her sleep and hot flash daily interference. Her progress is summarized and her complete daily diary and measures are provided as an example for comparison with your progress.

Hot Flash Score

For her fifth week of listening to the hypnosis recordings (three to six times) and using self-hypnosis four to five times a day, Emily reported a total of 21 hot flashes for the week, *all* of them falling into the mild/moderate columns of severity, indicating a dramatic shift in terms of severity and in the number of hot flashes reported.

Mild:	8 hot flashes	$\times\, 1 =$	8
Moderate:	13 hot flashes	$\times\, 2 =$	26
Severe:	0 hot flashes	$\times\, 3 =$	0
Very severe:	0 hot flashes	$\times\, 4 =$	0

34 = Emily's Week 5 Hot Flash Score

Reduction Percentage

Step 1: Subtract the current week's hot flash score from the baseline hot flash score.

146	Emily's baseline hot flash score
– 34	Emily's Week 5 hot flash score
112	Difference

Step 2: Divide the difference by the baseline hot flash score.

$112/146 = .77$

Step 3: Multiply the quotient times 100 to determine the percentage of decrease.

.77 × 100 = 77%

This reflects a decrease of 115 points in her hot flash score, or approximately a 77% reduction since her baseline recordings! Also, it is noteworthy that Emily has not had night sweats for *two weeks!*

Sleep

In chapter 9, I included Emily's baseline Sleep Rating Form, and based on her responses I feel comfortable saying her sleep quality was poor before she began hypnotic relaxation practice. One particular area that Emily reported a serious problem with was on the questions, "I went to sleep quickly," and "I stayed asleep most of the night," where she marked 2 and 0, respectively, indicating the answer, "not at all." In our discussions, she attributed this to anxiety that kept her from falling asleep and night sweats that woke her during the night. None of Emily's responses were beyond "4" on the 0 to 10 scale (0—not at all; 10—very much).

On page 206 you can see Emily's Sleep Rating Form after practicing hypnotic relaxation for these five weeks. Emily practiced daily for the first three weeks of the program and then three to six times a week thereafter with the recordings. She also began using self-hypnosis (without the recordings) beginning in the third week, and she reported to me that she often used self-hypnosis four to five times a day.

What a change! As you can see, Emily's sleep quality has improved tremendously. In our discussions, she described herself as "a normal person again" because of her ability to go to bed and fall asleep, sleep all night, and wake refreshed and feeling good in the morning.

She stated that people in her life commented on how her physical appearance had changed and she looked so much younger and happier!

Mood, Relationships, and Quality of Life

Emily's change from her baseline assessment of her HFRDIS scores to her postsessions assessment showed that she had achieved an improvement in her QOL that was remarkable. Hot flashes were no longer a source of interference in her life.

Please take a moment and look over Emily's Hot Flash Daily Diary, Hypnotic Relaxation Practice Checklist, Sleep Rating Form, and HFRDIS completed after her five weeks of practice of hypnotic relaxation. I think you would agree with me if I said she did great!

Emily's Week 5
HOT FLASH DAILY DIARY

| Date | Make a mark for each hot flash to indicate mild, moderate, severe, or very severe | | | | Total # of Hot Flashes Today | NOTES (Use this space to record possible triggers or other information relating to trends you may notice about your hot flashes) |
	MILD	MODE-RATE	SEVERE	VERY SEVERE		
MON 8/27/xx	I	II			3	Had 2 moderate ones while shopping—store was VERY crowded
TUES 8/28/xx	II	II			4	
WEDS 8/29/xx	II	II			4	
THURS 8/30/xx		II			2	
FRI 9/1/xx	I	II			3	
SAT 9/2/xx	I	I			2	
SUN 9/3/xx	I	II			3	
TOTALS	8	13			21	Had a VERY GOOD week!!!!

Severity Descriptors

Mild	Lasts <5 minutes; uncomfortable warmth; mild discomfort; no need for action
Moderate	Up to 15 minutes; warm, clammy skin; increased heart rate; some sweating; agitated; embarrassed; use fan, remove clothes, etc.
Severe	Up to 20 minutes; very hot; increased heart rate; unusual sensation over skin; sweating; anxiety; embarrassment; activity interruption
Very severe	Up to 45 minutes; extreme heat; rolling perspiration; increased heart rate; nausea; extreme distress; difficulty functioning; need to take cold shower or hold ice on skin

Emily's Week 5
HYPNOTIC RELAXATION
PRACTICE CHECKLIST

DATE: 9/2/xx

Week #:   ○ 1   ○ 2   ○ 3   ○ 4   ⊘ 5

1. *During the past week,* how often have you practiced hypnotic relaxation with the audio recording?

    Daily (seven times per week) or more   ☐

    Three to six times per week   ☒

    One to two times per week   ☐

    None   ☐

2. Please rate your average relaxation before hypnotic relaxation (Pre- session average):

    0   1   2   3   4   5   6   7   ⑧   9   10
    No   Extremely
    relaxation   relaxed

3. Please rate your average relaxation after hypnotic relaxation (Post- session average):

    0   1   2   3   4   5   6   7   8   9   ⑩
    No   Extremely
    relaxation   relaxed

Emily's Week 6
SLEEP RATING FORM

DATE: 9/2/xx

During the past week, about how many hours did you sleep each night on average? 7

Circle the number that best represents your agreement with the following comments regarding your sleep *during the past week*.

	Not at all										Very much so
1. I was relaxed during my sleep.	0	1	2	3	4	5	6	7	8	9	(10)
2. I went to sleep quickly.	0	1	2	3	4	5	6	7	8	(9)	10
3. My sleep was good.	0	1	2	3	4	5	6	7	8	(9)	10
4. I awoke very few times during the night.	0	1	2	3	4	5	6	7	8	(9)	10
5. For my age, I felt like I got an adequate amount of sleep.	0	1	2	3	4	5	6	7	8	9	(10)
6. I was satisfied with my sleep.	0	1	2	3	4	5	6	7	8	(9)	10
7. My sleep met my expectations.	0	1	2	3	4	5	6	7	8	(9)	10
8. I was able to go to sleep without sleeping pills or drugs.	0	1	2	3	4	5	6	7	8	9	(10)
9. I stayed asleep most of the night.	0	1	2	3	4	5	6	7	8	(9)	10
10. I woke up feeling refreshed.	0	1	2	3	4	5	6	7	8	9	(10)

TOTAL SCORE: 94

("I slept well": 0 = not at all; 100 = very much so)

Emily's Week 6
HOT FLASH RELATED DAILY
INTERFERENCE SCALE (HFRDIS)

DATE: 9/2/xx

Circle the number that best describes how much hot flashes have interfered with each aspect of your life during the past week.

	Not at all										Very much so
1. Work (work outside the home and house work)	(0)	1	2	3	4	5	6	7	8	9	10
2. Social activities (time spent with family, friends, etc.)	0	(1)	2	3	4	5	6	7	8	9	10
3. Leisure activities (time spent relaxing, doing hobbies, etc.)	(0)	1	2	3	4	5	6	7	8	9	10
4. Sleep	(0)	1	2	3	4	5	6	7	8	9	10
5. Mood	0	1	(2)	3	4	5	6	7	8	9	10
6. Concentration	0	1	(2)	3	4	5	6	7	8	9	10
7. Relations with others	0	(1)	2	3	4	5	6	7	8	9	10
8. Sexuality	(0)	1	2	3	4	5	6	7	8	9	10
9. Enjoyment of life	(0)	1	2	3	4	5	6	7	8	9	10
10. Overall quality of life	(0)	1	2	3	4	5	6	7	8	9	10

TOTAL SCORE: _6_

("Hot flashes interfered with my life": 0 = not at all; 100 = very much so)

IN THE WEEKS AHEAD

After you have completed your rating scales to assess sleep and hot flash interference affecting mood, relationships, and QOL as you perceive them after five weeks of hypnotic relaxation therapy practice, I think you will be truly amazed at your own progress! It is important that you continue your practice of hypnotic relaxation on a daily basis. You will probably need to do this for several more months to maintain your progress. Now that you know how to use hypnotic relaxation to reduce your hot flashes, it is important that you make it a part of your daily life so that you put your knowledge into good practice. You can also continue to keep your Hot Flash Daily Diary if you wish to further record your change.

It is possible that you have not seen results from this program that you had hoped to achieve. Perhaps you don't feel that your hot flashes have decreased in a way that you expected, or you are still having a really difficult time with your practices and in relaxing. There is hope! The next chapter addresses the most common challenges and provides suggestions to overcoming them.

Chapter 18

If You Need Additional Help

fter completing the five weeks of the *Relief from Hot Flashes* program and using hypnotic relaxation you have probably reduced your hot flashes pretty significantly. Most women who have completed the program report feeling fairly satisfied with their progress. But what if you are still having hot flashes? What should you do? First, look over your daily diaries and other measures to see where you need additional help. In this chapter, I will discuss the most common issues that can interfere with successfully reducing hot flashes, sleeping better, and reducing stress. Also, I will include some resources to consider if you need professional help from a health care provider with expertise in hypnotic relaxation therapy.

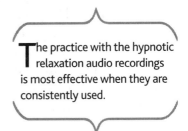

The practice with the hypnotic relaxation audio recordings is most effective when they are consistently used.

REGULAR PRACTICE WITH AUDIO RECORDINGS

One of the most important aspects of the program is to use the audio recordings on a daily basis. The practice with the audio recordings is most effective when they are consistently used and when you find the best times to practice. For some women the practice needs to be at night before going to sleep, but if that is not effective for you, then daytime practice is likely to be needed.

If you have had something happen that has interfered with you being able to use the audio recordings in the most effective manner, then you may need to make some adjustments. For example, one of my patients was playing the audio recordings on her laptop computer, but she had a problem with being able to effectively use it because it was cumbersome to use in the bedroom and sometimes her son wanted to use the laptop. In her case, she was able to put the recordings on a CD and bought an inexpensive CD player that was battery-operated, allowing her to take it with her and use the audio recordings of hypnotic relaxation in a way that was very convenient.

FINDING A SAFE PLACE TO PRACTICE

Finding a good place to practice hypnotic relaxation can sometimes be a challenge. In the course of a busy day, it is not always easy to find a safe and quiet environment where you can spend about 30 minutes in a hypnotic state of relaxation. If this has been difficult, I would suggest you discuss with your family a plan that would provide you with more support and ensure the protected time needed to practice hypnotic relaxation. It may be that you need to talk with friends or coworkers to find some ideas for accommodating you, or you may need to just be more assertive in expressing your needs! Please recognize that no one can practice hypnotic relaxation without feeling they are in a safe environment where they will not be interrupted for that brief period of time.

REVIEW ANY TRIGGERS

It has been noted that some of the issues that can affect hot flashes are the influence of stress and circumstances that may serve as triggers. For example, if you have had something very stressful happen since you began the program, it may have affected your progress. Review the forms in which you noted triggers and you may identify some circumstances or stressors that you need to address before you resume your practice of hypnotic relaxation on a daily basis.

MAINTAIN A HOT FLASH DAILY DIARY

Consistently maintaining a Hot Flash Daily Diary is essential to your success. Before actually starting hypnotic relaxation, you began the program by recording a full week of hot flashes. Recording all of the hot flashes and rating their severity was very important to track your progress and to help guide your subsequent practice of hypnotic relaxation.

Maintaining a Hot Flash Daily Diary takes some time, and keeping the diary with you so that you can write down all of the hot flashes that occur may be a little inconvenient. Everyone's life is busy and I have attempted to minimize the burden of keeping the diary so that just a mark is needed to record hot flash events. I know that even that takes time, but you need to remember to do it. Keeping a Hot Flash Daily Diary throughout the program and recording your hot flashes accurately and consistently is important. After you have completed the program and have reduced your hot flashes to a satisfactory level, you will no longer need to continue to keep the diary.

IDENTIFICATION OF INDIVIDUALIZED MENTAL IMAGERY

Finding the best individualized mental imagery for coolness and relaxation also can be very important in reducing hot flashes. For some women the personal imagery is something that relates to a past vacation or a situation that they relate to as free of stress and bringing feelings of coolness. It may relate to a time in childhood or another time in your life. The individualized mental imagery should relate to something that you have actually experienced—something that you feel very good about, and about which you have good memories.

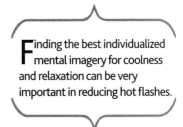

Finding the best individualized mental imagery for coolness and relaxation can be very important in reducing hot flashes.

In the practice of hypnotic relaxation for reducing hot flashes, you were asked to identify some personal imagery that has a strong and very positive emotional resonance for you and might help you to achieve a hypnotic state and a sense of coolness. If an individualized mental image does not bring about good and positive emotion, coolness, and relaxation, then you should identify some other mental imagery, or simply allow yourself to notice whatever images spontaneously come into your mind as you drift into a deeper hypnotic state while listening to one of the audio recordings.

EFFECTIVE USE OF SELF-HYPNOSIS

As you progressed through the program you began to learn the methods of self-hypnosis. For many women this is an essential part of the program and is very empowering. However, it does require active involvement and dedicated use of the techniques. It is important that you are doing *both* self-hypnosis and using the audio recordings. The frequency of self-hypnosis practice depends on the needs of the individual. Some women find that they need to practice once a day and others as many as ten times a day. Also, by reviewing your triggers for hot flashes you may identify times to practice self-hypnosis that will be most effective for you.

DON'T TRY TOO HARD

Another issue that some women have encountered is whether or not to use headphones. Headphones or ear buds work very well to help block out distractions and allow you to practice hypnotic relaxation even if there is someone else in the room (such as a bed partner at night). However, headphones can themselves be uncomfortable when going to sleep. Some women have found that placing the headphones on the pillow, very near their ears, is an effective way to listen to the recordings.

Earlier in this book I discussed some of the principles of hypnotic suggestion. With hypnotic relaxation, it is important to strive for an accepting attitude of "letting go" and allowing a relaxed hypnotic state to occur. Trying too hard can interfere with progress. This is a common problem with highly motivated individuals who find it hard to "let go" and just relax, but with practice and understanding it is within the grasp of everyone!

PERSISTENCE PAYS OFF

The phrase "persistence pays off" can help you remain confident that your hot flashes will lessen. As other women have been able to reduce their hot flashes, with the right conditions, so will you. In the research on hypnotic relaxation for hot flashes it has been shown that the five-week program works well for the vast majority of women. However, I have had some women who have needed additional weeks of practice to achieve the same results. There is no way to predict in advance exactly how many sessions you will need. It can only be discovered by practice and experience. Don't give up, if your hot flashes are not reduced to where you want them to be, continuing the program may provide the help you need.

STRESS AND EMOTIONAL FACTORS

Stress and emotional factors can also affect progress with hypnotic relaxation. In addition to serving as hot flash triggers, you may be experiencing more significant stress or even depression. Stress and emotional factors can be connected to a major change at work or in your relationships, marital problems, a death in the family, depression, a history of anxiety, or significant financial issues. If you are overly worried, depressed, or distressed about something, it will be difficult to concentrate and relax. Sometimes during the practice of hypnotic relaxation, a woman becomes aware that she is dealing with depression, anxiety, or even post-traumatic stress. If that is the case, a mental health care provider should by consulted to get the help needed.

PROFESSIONAL HELP

This book and its accompanying audio recordings provide all of the tools you need to use hypnotic relaxation to reduce your hot flashes, but you may find it helpful to have a trained professional guide you through the weekly sessions or to practice in combination with counseling. This can be accomplished by consulting with a clinical psychologist, nurse, physician, or other mental health care provider with expertise in hypnotherapy and hypnotic relaxation.

Fortunately there are some very good organizations that you can turn to in order to find a professional with expertise in hypnotic relaxation–based methods. These organizations typically include licensed health care providers in the fields of medicine, psychology, nursing, social work, professional counseling, or complementary areas that use hypnotherapy. Leading organizations in the United States include the following.

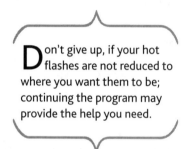

Don't give up, if your hot flashes are not reduced to where you want them to be; continuing the program may provide the help you need.

American Society of Clinical Hypnosis (ASCH)

www.asch.net

ASCH is a primary organization in the United States for clinical practitioners including physicians, psychologists, mental health counselors, social workers, nurse practitioners, dentists, and chiropractors who use hypnotherapy. ASCH also has a certification program in clinical hypnosis for qualified health care providers. The website includes a member referral search for practitioners in your area.

Society for Clinical and Experimental Hypnosis (SCEH)

www.sceh.us

SCEH is the leading organization for both clinical and experimental hypnosis. The society publishes the *International Journal of Clinical and Experimental Hypnosis* and maintains a certification listing.

Society for Psychological Hypnosis (Division 30 of the American Psychological Association)

www.psychologicalhypnosis.com

Members include psychologists and other health care providers and scientists with an interest in clinical and experimental hypnosis.

International Society of Hypnosis (ISH)

www.ish-hypnosis.org

An international organization with component societies from around the world, including Australia, Canada, Denmark, Germany, France, Mexico, and the United Kingdom.

Canadian Society of Hypnosis (CSH)

www.hypnosis.bc.ca

CSH includes component societies from across Canada. It is a leading organization to find qualified health care providers with expertise in hypnosis in Canada.

Afterword: Women Share Their Experiences Using the *Relief from Hot Flashes* Program

This section is included to provide you with some ideas of how other women have used the program and what they have found effective for them. I hope you enjoy reading how Sally, Mary, and Linda reduced their hot flashes and planned for the future. Best wishes for your future as well!

SALLY

How did you find out about hypnotic relaxation therapy?

My husband found an article in the newspaper about this program and brought it to me. He wanted me to try it. My husband went to great lengths to help me with my hot flashes.

What was your reaction to the idea of hypnosis?

I was excited and intrigued. I'm not the kind of person looking for "here is the pill, take it." I was looking for a more natural way to deal with my hot flashes. The thought of a natural process to get control of my hot flashes was just so appealing to me. I recognize there's a stigma attached to the word "hypnosis." People think it's about making someone bark like a dog. That's not what it really is.

How would you describe a session?

It's like a spa. It's wonderful. It's my time. It's my "me" time. Sometimes I have trouble calling it hypnosis because you're just helping us relax our own bodies. Yes, we are visualizing something to help calm us down, but you're not really suggesting that we do something that we wouldn't normally do. To me it's really just relaxation and helping you get control over your own body.

In addition to a reduction in your hot flashes, what benefits have you experienced?

The visualization is great, it really is, but teaching me to relax one muscle, one body part at a time, is just amazing. Hypnotic relaxation therapy is a great tool to help in every aspect of your life, not just the hot flashes. It helps me in so many ways, like in stress relief at work and at home. It's wonderful.

What components of therapy stood out to you?

The absolute euphoria when you wake up. You feel rested and relaxed. It's 30 minutes and you could have slept for 10 hours.

MARY

Had you considered hormone replacement therapy to treat your hot flashes?

I was just getting ready to try hormone replacement therapy when the media started reporting on the side effects it had on women's bodies. Breast cancer runs in my family and it was reported that if you're prone to breast cancer, hormone replacement therapy could cause some problems. And I thought, I don't want to do this if I don't have to. So when I learned about hypnotic relaxation therapy on the news, I wanted to talk to my doctor about it. At my next appointment, I said, "You know, let me try this first." I almost saw him roll his eyes. He said, "You can try this if you want to, but we should set you up an appointment in a couple of months and we can talk more about hormone replacement then." I thought, I'm going to show you, I'm going to try this.

I waited until I went through the whole program to go back to him. When I did, I gave him a couple of brochures and a magazine article and I told him to read up on it because it worked for me.

What was your reaction to the idea of hypnosis?

I always tell people I do relaxation therapy because that seems to have a little better response than hypnosis. They understand relaxation therapy; a lot of them don't understand hypnosis. Because hypnosis does have kind of a carnival-vibe based on the way it's presented.

How would you describe a session?

You go to a place in your mind that's going to cool you off. It's almost like your body is cooling itself off.

What surprised you about hypnosis?

I was surprised that you don't go completely under. I thought I was going to be put completely under and I wasn't going to remember anything that happened to me or know what I was doing. But you do know exactly what you're doing. You're conscious of everything that you're doing. You're aware of everything that is happening to you. You always have control. And that's what I wanted, to get control of my own body.

What was your reaction when you felt your hot flashes decreasing?

I was very, very grateful because I had between 15 and 17 hot flashes a day. And I still have them, but now it's two or three. Sometimes I go days without them. I don't have night sweats anymore.

Describe your experience with self-hypnosis.

You don't realize how much you can do on your own until you are given the tools. Most of the time, my self-hypnosis lasts less than a minute. I've done it enough so it doesn't take me very long at all. If I have 30 to 45 seconds by myself, I can talk myself out of a hot flash.

When did the hot flashes start to decrease?

Mine decreased as time went on. I think at my last session I was down to four or five a day. And they've even gone down below that now. I listen to the audio recordings each night and do self-hypnosis when I feel a hot flash coming on. If I'm at work, I'll just go off alone and put myself in a little trance and talk to myself for a minute and then they go away and I'm fine. And there are days that I don't have any.

In addition to a reduction in your hot flashes, what benefits have you experienced?

It helps me control my body temperature. For me, experiencing a hot flash felt like somebody had a dimmer switch and they put that dimmer switch all the way up to high. With hypnotic relaxation therapy that dimmer switch doesn't go all the way up to the top. I have the control. It's also a great stress reliever. I can control my stress level now, too.

What would you say to someone who is skeptical of this therapy?

Put aside your preconceived notions about hypnosis and give it a chance. I have a younger sister who is just starting to experience hot flashes and I told her, "I'm going to make a copy of the audio files and send them to you. You really need to listen to these." And I think she will. I think she'll be able to follow the program. If she gives it a try.

LINDA

Did you speak to your doctor about hypnotic relaxation therapy?

I did, and he was really encouraging. He said, "Let me know how it goes." He was really open to it.

What was your reaction to the idea of hypnosis?

I had two friends that used it and for one of them it cut the hot flashes in half. So I knew it worked. I was open to it and I think that's what made it work like it did for me. I was never embarrassed to tell anybody I was doing it because it's something that's working for me, so it doesn't matter.

When do you practice?

Right before I go to bed. It helps me fall asleep. I also do little sessions because I don't have time at work to do the whole thing. But if I feel like I'm getting stressed, I'll do a mini-session and that's helped me a lot.

How important was the individualization of imagery to you?

It made a big difference. The imagery was my own. It was mine and not for anybody else. It wasn't "this is what everybody does, you try and do the same, you try to fit into this mold." It was "what do you want this to be?"

When did you hot flashes start to decrease?

After the second or third session.

How did you feel when you felt your hot flashes decreasing?

Great, especially when the night sweats stopped for me. I listened to the audio recordings right before I went to bed and they just stopped. I was able to sleep through the night. And that's great. Night sweats are horrible. You can't get away from the heat at all.

In addition to a reduction in your hot flashes, what benefits have you experienced?

The stress relief is amazing. I feel so absolutely relaxed it is unbelievable.

I like that we get back control of our bodies. Control is the key thing. You can control your body, your temperature, your attitude, anything, you can control it. And that's what I was missing. You don't have to go through a hot flash. You can actually stop it and make it go away.

Describe your experience with self-hypnosis.

It's like you're talking yourself out of a hot flash. Whenever I get stressed or feel a hot flash coming on, I try to use it. The self-hypnosis helped me a lot. I used the audio recordings every night, but I use the self-hypnosis almost every day.

How would you describe hypnotic relaxation therapy to others?

It's like another form of relaxation, that's all it is. I would tell them, "The therapist gives you suggestions to relax you and calm your-self down. And you are aware, you are not asleep. You can hear the therapist talking. You go into a very relaxed state of mind. And when you finish your session you feel great."

If you could tell other women about your experience, what would you say?

I would say to try it, give into it, and be open to it, because it does work. I thought I couldn't do it, but you can do it and you'll start looking forward to it.

Appendix

The following pages provide blank copies of the five forms used to chart your progress throughout the *Relief from Hot Flashes* program

Hot Flash Daily Diary
Hot Flash Triggers log
Sleep Rating Form
Hot Flash Related Daily Interference Scale (HFRDIS)
and the Hypnotic Relaxation Practice Checklist

You can copy the forms provided here or download digital copies of the forms from www.demoshealth.com/store/elkins-relief-from-hot-flashes-supplements

HOT FLASH DAILY DIARY

Date	Make a mark for each hot flash to indicate mild, moderate, severe, or very severe				Total # of Hot Flashes Today	NOTES (Use this space to record possible triggers or other information relating to trends you may notice about your hot flashes)
	MILD	MODE-RATE	SEVERE	VERY SEVERE		
MON / /						
TUES / /						
WEDS / /						
THURS / /						
FRI / /						
SAT / /						
SUN / /						
TOTALS						

Severity Descriptors

Mild	Lasts <5 minutes; uncomfortable warmth; mild discomfort; no need for action
Moderate	Up to 15 minutes; warm, clammy skin; increased heart rate; some sweating; agitated; embarrassed; use fan, remove clothes, etc.
Severe	Up to 20 minutes; very hot; increased heart rate; unusual sensation over skin; sweating; anxiety; embarrassment; activity interruption
Very severe	Up to 45 minutes; extreme heat; rolling perspiration; increased heart rate; nausea; extreme distress; difficulty functioning; need to take cold shower or hold ice on skin

HOT FLASH TRIGGERS

POTENTIAL TRIGGER	ACTIVITY

SLEEP RATING FORM

DATE: _____

During the past week, about how many hours did you sleep each night on average? _____

Circle the number that best represents your agreement with the following comments regarding your sleep *during the past week.*

	Not at all									Very much so
1. I was relaxed during my sleep.	0	1	2	3	4	5	6	7	8	9	10
2. I went to sleep quickly.	0	1	2	3	4	5	6	7	8	9	10
3. My sleep was good.	0	1	2	3	4	5	6	7	8	9	10
4. I awoke very few times during the night.	0	1	2	3	4	5	6	7	8	9	10
5. For my age, I felt like I got an adequate amount of sleep.	0	1	2	3	4	5	6	7	8	9	10
6. I was satisfied with my sleep.	0	1	2	3	4	5	6	7	8	9	10
7. My sleep met my expectations.	0	1	2	3	4	5	6	7	8	9	10
8. I was able to go to sleep without sleeping pills or drugs.	0	1	2	3	4	5	6	7	8	9	10
9. I stayed asleep most of the night.	0	1	2	3	4	5	6	7	8	9	10
10. I woke up feeling refreshed.	0	1	2	3	4	5	6	7	8	9	10

TOTAL SCORE: _____

("I slept well": 0 = not at all; 100 = very much so)

HOT FLASH RELATED DAILY INTERFERENCE SCALE (HFRDIS)

DATE: _____

Circle the number that best describes how much hot flashes have interfered with each aspect of your life *during the past week*.

	Not at all										Very much so
1. Work (work outside the home and house work)	0	1	2	3	4	5	6	7	8	9	10
2. Social activities (time spent with family, friends, etc.)	0	1	2	3	4	5	6	7	8	9	10
3. Leisure activities (time spent relaxing, doing hobbies, etc.)	0	1	2	3	4	5	6	7	8	9	10
4. Sleep	0	1	2	3	4	5	6	7	8	9	10
5. Mood	0	1	2	3	4	5	6	7	8	9	10
6. Concentration	0	1	2	3	4	5	6	7	8	9	10
7. Relations with others	0	1	2	3	4	5	6	7	8	9	10
8. Sexuality	0	1	2	3	4	5	6	7	8	9	10
9. Enjoyment of life	0	1	2	3	4	5	6	7	8	9	10
10. Overall quality of life	0	1	2	3	4	5	6	7	8	9	10

TOTAL SCORE: _____

("Hot flashes interfered with my life": 0 = not at all; 100 = very much so)

HYPNOTIC RELAXATION
PRACTICE CHECKLIST

DATE: _____

Week #: ○ 1   ○ 2   ○ 3   ○ 4   ○ 5

1. *During the past week,* how often have you practiced hypnotic relaxation with the audio recording?

Daily (seven times per week) or more	☐
Three to six times per week	☐
One to two times per week	☐
None	☐

2. Please rate your average relaxation before hypnotic relaxation (Presession average):

0   1   2   3   4   5   6   7   8   9   10
No   Extremely
relaxation   relaxed

3. Please rate your average relaxation after hypnotic relaxation (Postsession average):

0   1   2   3   4   5   6   7   8   9   10
No   Extremely
relaxation   relaxed

Bibliography

PREFACE

Elkins, G., Fisher, W., Johnson, A., Carpenter, J. S., & Keith, T. Z. (2013). Clinical hypnosis in the treatment of postmenopausal hot flashes: A randomized controlled trial. *Menopause, 20*(3), 291–298 (Original work published 2012).

Elkins, G., Marcus, J., Palamara, L., & Stearns, V. (2004). Can hypnosis reduce hot flashes in breast cancer survivors? A literature review. *American Journal of Clinical Hypnosis, 47*(1), 29–42.

Elkins, G., Marcus, J., Stearns, V., Perfect, M., Rajab, M. H., Ruud, C., … Keith, T. (2008). Randomized trial of a hypnosis intervention for treatment of hot flashes among breast cancer survivors. *Journal of Clinical Oncology, 26*(31), 5022–5026.

Elkins, G., Stearns, V., Marcus, J., & Rajab, H. (2007). Pilot evaluation of hypnosis for treatment of hot flashes in breast cancer survivors. *Psycho-Oncology, 16*(5), 487–492.

CHAPTER 1

Bachmann, G. A. (1999). Vasomotor flushes in menopausal women. *American Journal of Obstetrics and Gynecology, 180*(3), 312–316.

Carpenter, J. S. (2005a). State of the science: Hot flashes and cancer, part 1: Definition, scope, impact, physiology, and measurement. *Oncology Nursing Forum, 32*(5), 959–968.

Carpenter, J. S. (2005b). State of the science: Hot flashes and cancer, part 2: Management and future directions. *Oncology Nursing Forum, 32*(5), 969–978.

Carpenter, J. S., Andrykowski, M. A., Cordova, M., Cunningham, L., Studts, J., McGrath, P., … Munn, R. (1998). Hot flashes in postmenopausal women treated for breast carcinoma: Prevalence, severity, correlates, management, and relation to quality of life. *Cancer, 82*(9), 1682–1691.

Elkins, G., Fisher, W. I., Johnson, A. K., Carpenter, J. S., & Keith, T. Z. (2013). Clinical hypnosis in the treatment of postmenopausal hot flashes: A randomized controlled trial. *Menopause, 20*(3), 291–298. (Epub ahead of print Oct. 22. 2012 PMID: 23096250).

Elkins, G., Johnson, A., Fisher, W., Sliwinski, J., & Keith, T. (2013) A pilot investigation of guided self-hypnosis in the treatment of hot flashes among postmenopausal women. *International Journal of Clinical and Experimental Hypnosis, 61*(3), 342–350.

Elkins, G., Marcus, J, Stearns, V., Perfect, M., Rajab, M. H., Ruud, C., ... Keith, T. (2008). Randomized trial of a hypnosis intervention for treatment of hot flashes among breast cancer survivors. *Journal of Clinical Oncology, 26*(31), 5022–5026.

Elkins, G. R., Marcus, J., Bunn, J., Perfect, M., Palamara, L., Stearns, V., & Dove, J. (2010). Preferences for hypnotic imagery for hot flash reduction: A brief communication. *International Journal of Clinical and Experimental Hypnosis, 58*(3), 345–349.

Kronenberg, F. (1990). Hot flashes: Epidemiology and physiology. *Annals of the New York Academy of Sciences, 592*(1), 52–86.

North American Menopause Society. (2012). *The menopause guidebook.* Mayfield Heights, OH: Author.

Stearns, V., Ullmer, L., Lopez, J. F., Smith, Y., Isaacs, C., & Hayes, D. (2002). Hot flushes. *The Lancet, 360*(9348), 1851–1861.

Stein, K. D., Jacobsen, P. B., Hann, D. M., Greenberg, H., & Lyman, G. (2000). Impact of hot flashes on quality of life among postmenopausal women being treated for breast cancer. *Journal of Pain and Symptom Management, 19*(6), 436–445.

CHAPTER 2

Barrett, K., Barman, S., Boitano, S., & Heddwen, B. (2012) *Gonong's Review of Medical Physiology* (24th ed.), New York, NY: McGraw-Hill Medical

Carpenter, J. S., Monahan, P. O., & Azzouz, F. (2004). Accuracy of subjective hot flush reports compared with continuous sternal skin conductance monitoring. *Obstetrics and Gynecology, 104*(6), 1322–1326.

Freedman, R. R., & Blacker, C. M. (2002). Estrogen raises the sweating threshold in postmenopausal women with hot flashes. *Fertility and Sterility, 77*(3), 487–490.

Freedman, R. R., & Krell, W. (1999). Reduced thermoregulatory null zone in postmenopausal women with hot flashes. *American Journal of Obstetrics and Gynecology, 181*(1), 66–70.

Freeman, E. W., Sammel, M. D., Lin, H., Gracia, C. R., Kapoor, S., & Ferdousi, T. (2005). The role of anxiety and hormonal changes in menopausal hot flashes. *Menopause 12*(3), 258–266.

Gannon, L., Hansel, S., & Goodwin, J. (1987). Correlates of menopausal hot flashes. *Journal of Behavioral Medicine, 10*(3), 277–285.

Kronenberg, F. (1994). Hot flashes: Phenomenology, quality of life, and search for treatment options. *Experimental Gerontology, 29*(3/4), 319–336.

Stearns, V., Ulmer, L., Lopez, J. F., Smith, Y., Isaacs, C., & Hayes, D. (2002). Hot flushes. *The Lancet, 360*, 1851–1861.

Swartzman, L. C., Edelberg, R., & Kemmann, E. (1990). Impact of stress on objectively recorded menopausal hot flushes and on flush report bias. *Health Psychology, 9*, 529–545.

Voda, A. M. (1981). Climacteric hot flash. *Maturitas, 3*(1), 73–90.

CHAPTER 3

Baum, A. & Anderson, B. L. (2001). *Psychosocial interventions for cancer*. Washington, DC : American Psychological Association.

Carpenter, J. S., Andrykowski, M. A., Cordova, M., Cunningham, L., Studts, J., McGrath, P., ... Munn, R. (1998). Hot flashes in post menopausal women treated for breast carcinoma: Prevalence, severity, correlates, management, and relation to quality of life. *Cancer, 82*, 1682–1691.

Derogatis, L. R. Morrow, G. R., Fetting, J., Penman, D. Piasetsky, S., Schmale, A. M., ... Carnike, C. L., Jr. (1983). The prevalence of psychiatric disorders among cancer patients. *Journal of the American Medical Association, 249*, 751–757.

Elkins, G. R., Jensen, M., & Patterson, D. (2007). Hypnotherapy for the management of chronic pain. *International Journal of Clinical and Experimental Hypnosis, 55*(3), 275–287.

Elkins, G. R., Marcus, J, Stearns, V., Perfect, M., Rajab, M. H., Ruud, C., ... Keith, T. (2008). Randomized trial of a hypnosis intervention for treatment of hot flashes among breast cancer survivors. *Journal of Clinical Oncology, 26*(31), 5022–5026.

Elkins, G. R., Perfect, M., & Ruud, C. (2008). Biobehavioral treatment of hot flashes in a 48-year-old menopausal woman. In R. Kessler & D. Stafford (Eds.), *Collaborative medicine case studies: Evidence in practice* (pp. 177–185). New York, NY: Springer Publishing.

Elkins, G. R., Stearns, V., Marcus, J., & Rajab, H. (2007). Pilot evaluation of hypnosis for treatment of hot flashes in breast cancer survivors. *Psycho-Oncology, 16*(5), 487–492.

Holland, J. C., Greenberg, D. B., & Hughes, M. K. (2006) *Quick reference for oncology clinicians: The psychiatric and psychosocial dimensions of cancer symptom management*. Charlottesville, VA: American Psychosocial Oncology Society.

Irvine, D., Brown, B., Crooks, D., Roberts, J., & Browne, G. (1991). Psychosocial adjustment in women with breast cancer. *Cancer, 67*, 1097–1117.

Labriola, D. (2000). *Complementary cancer therapies*. Roseville, CA: Prima Health: A Division of Prima Publishing.

Spiegel, D. (1993). *Living beyond limits: New help and hope for facing life-threatening illness*. New York, NY: Times Books/Random House.

Spiegel, D., & Bloom, J. R. (1983). Group therapy and hypnosis to reduce metastatic breast carcinoma pain. *Psychosomatic Medicine, 45*, 333–339.

Vinokur, A. D., Threatt, B. A., Caplan, R. D., & Zimmerman, B. L. (1989). Physical and psychosocial functioning and adjustment to breast cancer: Long-term follow-up of a screen population. *Cancer, 63*, 394–405.

CHAPTER 4

Abdali, K., Khajehei, M., & Tabatabaee, H. R. (2010). Effect of St John's wort on severity, frequency, and duration of hot flashes in premenopausal, perimenopausal and postmenopausal women: A randomized, double-blind, placebo-controlled study. *Menopause, 17*(2), 326–331.

Aguirre, W., Chedraui, P., Mendoza, J., & Ruilova, I. (2010). Gabapentin vs. low-dose transdermal estradiol for treating post menopausal women with moderate to very severe hot flushes. *Gynecological Endocrinology, 26*(5), 333–337.

Aiello, E. J., Yasui, Y., Tworoger, S. S., Ulrich, C. M., Irwin, M. L., Bowen, D., … McTiernan, A. (2004). Effect of a yearlong, moderate-intensity exercise intervention on the occurrence and severity of menopause symptoms in postmenopausal women. *Menopause, 11*(4), 382–388.

American College of Obstetricians and Gynecologists Committee on Gynecologic Practice. (2008). ACOG Committee Opinion No. 420, November 2008: Hormone therapy and heart disease. *Obstetrics and Gynecology, 112,* 1189–1192.

Anderson, G. L., Chlebowski, R. T., Rossouw, J. E., Rodabough, R. J., McTiernan, A., Margolis, K. L., … Ritenbaugh, C. (2006). Prior hormone therapy and breast cancer risk in the Women's Health Initiative randomized trial of estrogen plus progestin. *Maturitas, 55*(2), 103–115.

Anderson, G. L., Judd, H. L., Kaunitz, A. M., Barad, D. H., Beresford, S. A., Pettinger, M., … Lopez, A. M. (2003). Effects of estrogen plus progestin on gynecologic cancers and associated diagnostic procedures: The Women's Health Initiative Randomized trial. *JAMA, 290*(13), 1739–1748.

Barton, D., LaVasseur, B. I., Loprinzi, C., Novotny, P., Wilwerding, M. B., & Sloan, J. (2002). Venlafaxine for the control of hot flashes: Results of a longitudinal continuation study. *Oncology Nursing Forum, 29*(1), pp. 33–40.

Barton, D. L., LaVasseur, B. I., Sloan, J. A., Stawis, A. N., Flynn, K. A., Dyar, M., … Loprinzi, C. L. (2010). Phase III, placebo-controlled trial of three doses of citalopram for the treatment of hot flashes: NCCTG trial N05C9. *Journal of Clinical Oncology, 28*(20), 3278–3283.

Barton, D. L., Loprinzi, C. L., Quella, S. K., Sloan, J. A., Veeder, M. H., Egner, J. R., … Novotny, P. (1998). Prospective evaluation of vitamin E for hot flashes in breast cancer survivors. *Journal of Clinical Oncology, 16*(2), 495–500.

Bergmans, M. G. M., Merkus, J. M. W. M., Corbey, R. S., Schellekens, L. A., & Ubachs, J. M. H. (1987). Effect of Bellergal Retard on climacteric complaints: A double-blind, placebo-controlled study. *Maturitas, 9*(3), 227–234.

Boekhout, A. H., Vincent, A. D., Dalesio, O. B., van den Bosch, J., Foekema-Töns, J. H., Adriaansz, S., … Schellens, J. H. (2011). Management of hot flashes in patients who have breast cancer with venlafaxine and clonidine: A randomized, double-blind, placebo-controlled trial. *Journal of Clinical Oncology, 29*(29), 3862–3868.

Bolaños, R., Del Castillo, A., & Francia, J. (2010). Soy isoflavones versus placebo in the treatment of climacteric vasomotor symptoms: Systematic review and meta-analysis. *Menopause, 17*(3), 660–666.

Bonnick, S. L., Harris, S. T., Kendler, D. L., McClung, M. R., & Silverman, S. L. (2010). Management of osteoporosis in postmenopausal women: 2010 position statement of the North American Menopause Society. *Menopause, 17*(1), 25–54.

Butt, D. A., Lock, M., Lewis, J. E., Ross, S., & Moineddin, R. (2008). Gabapentin for the treatment of menopausal hot flashes: A randomized controlled trial. *Menopause, 15*(2), 310–318.

Carmody, J., Crawford, S., & Churchill, L. (2006). A pilot study of mindfulness-based stress reduction for hot flashes. *Menopause, 13*(5), 760–769.

Carmody, J., Crawford, S., Salmoirago-Blotcher, E., Leung, K., Churchill, L., & Olendzki, N. (2011). Mindfulness training for coping with hot flashes: Results of a randomized trial. *Menopause, 18*(6), 611–620.

Carpenter, J. S., Guthrie, K. A., Larson, J. C., Freeman, E. W., Joffe, H., Reed, S. D., ... LaCroix, A. Z. (2012). Effect of escitalopram on hot flash interference: A randomized, controlled trial. *Fertility and Sterility, 97*(6), 1399–1404.

Carpenter, J. S., Storniolo, A. M., Johns, S., Monahan, P. O., Azzouz, F., Elam, J. L., ... Shelton, R. C. (2007). Randomized, double-blind, placebo-controlled cross-over trials of venlafaxine for hot flashes after breast cancer. *The Oncologist, 12*(1), 124–135.

Carson, J. W., Carson, K. M., Porter, L. S., Keefe, F. J., & Seewaldt, V. L. (2009). Yoga of Awareness program for menopausal symptoms in breast cancer survivors: Results from a randomized trial. *Supportive Care in Cancer, 17*(10), 1301–1309.

Cauley, J. A., Robbins, J., Chen, Z., Cummings, S. R., Jackson, R. D., LaCroix, A. Z., ... Watts, N. B. (2003). Effects of estrogen plus progestin on risk of fracture and bone mineral density. *The Journal of the American Medical Association, 290*(13), 1729–1738.

Chlebowski, R. T., Hendrix, S. L., Langer, R. D., Stefanick, M. L., Gass, M., Lane, D., ... McTiernan, A. (2003). Influence of estrogen plus progestin on breast cancer and mammography in healthy postmenopausal women: the Women's Health Initiative randomized trial. *The Journal of the American Medical Association, 289*(24), 3243–3253.

Chlebowski, R. T., Wactawski-Wende, J., Ritenbaugh, C., Hubbell, F. A., Ascensao, J., Rodabough, R. J., ... White, E. (2004). Estrogen plus progestin and colorectal cancer in postmenopausal women. *The New England Journal of Medicine, 350*(10), 991–1004.

Christy, C. (1945). Vitamin E in menopause. *American Journal of Obstetrics and Gynecology, 50*(1), 84–87.

Clayden, J. R., Bell, J. W., & Pollard, P. (1974). Menopausal flushing: Double-blind trial of a non-hormonal medication. *British Medical Journal, 1*(5905), 409–412.

Col, N. F., Fairfield, K. M., Ewan-Whyte, C., & Miller, H. (2009). In the clinic. *Annals of Internal Medicine, 150*(7), 114–115.

Elavsky, S., Gonzales, J. U., Proctor, D. N., Williams, N., & Henderson, V. W. (2012). Effects of physical activity on vasomotor symptoms: Examination using objective and subjective measures. *Menopause, 19*(10), 1095–1103.

Evans, M. L., Pritts, E., Vittinghoff, E., McClish, K., Morgan, K. S., & Jaffe, R. B. (2005). Management of postmenopausal hot flushes with venlafaxine hydrochloride: A randomized, controlled trial. *Obstetrics and Gynecology, 105*(1), 161–166.

Freedman, R. R., & Woodward, S. (1992). Behavioral treatment of menopausal hot flushes: Evaluation by ambulatory monitoring. *American Journal of Obstetrics and Gynecology, 167*(2), 436–439.

Freedman, R. R., Woodward, S., Brown, B., Javaid, J. I., & Pandey, G. N. (1995). Biochemical and thermoregulatory effects of behavioral treatment for menopausal hot flashes. *Menopause, 2*(4), 211–218.

Freeman, E. W., Guthrie, K. A., Caan, B., Sternfeld, B., Cohen, L. S., Joffe, H., ... LaCroix, A. Z. (2011). Efficacy of escitalopram for hot flashes in healthy menopausal women: A randomized control trial. *The Journal of the American Medical Association, 305*(3), 267–274.

Gaweesh, S. S., Abdel-Gawad, M. M., Nagaty, A. M., & Ewies, A. A. (2010). Folic acid supplementation may cure hot flushes in postmenopausal women: A prospective cohort study. *Gynecological Endocrinology, 26*(9), 658–662.

Geller, S. E., Shulman, L. P., van Breemen, R. B., Banuvar, S., Zhou, Y., Epstein, G., ... Farnsworth, N. R. (2009). Safety and efficacy of black cohosh and red clover for the management of vasomotor symptoms: A randomized controlled trial. *Menopause, 16*(6), 1156–1166.

Geller, S. E., & Studee, L. (2005). Botanical and dietary supplements for menopausal symptoms: What works, what does not. *Journal of Women's Health, 14*(7), 634–649.

Germaine, L. M., & Freedman, R. R. (1984). Behavioral treatment of menopausal hot flashes: Evaluation by objective methods. *Journal of Consulting and Clinical Psychology, 52*(6), 1072–1079.

Goldberg, R. M., Loprinzi, C. L., O'Fallon, J. R., Veeder, M. H., Miser, A. W., Mailliard, J. A., ... Burnham, N. L. (1994). Transdermal clonidine for ameliorating tamoxifen-induced hot flashes. *Journal of Clinical Oncology, 12*(1), 155–158.

Goodwin, J. W., Green, S. J., Moinpour, C. M., Bearden, J. D., Giguere, J. K., Jiang, C. S., ... Albain, K. S. (2008). Phase III randomized placebo-controlled trial of two doses of megestrol acetate as treatment for menopausal symptoms in women with breast cancer: Southwest Oncology Group Study 9626. *Journal of Clinical Oncology, 26*(10), 1650–1656.

Gordon, P. R., Kerwin, J. P., Boesen, K. G., & Senf, J. (2006). Sertraline to treat hot flashes: A randomized controlled, double-blind, crossover trial in a general population. *Menopause, 13*(4), 568–575.

Guttuso, T., Jr., Kurlan, R., McDermott, M. P., & Kieburtz, K. (2003). Gabapentin's effects on hot flashes in postmenopausal women: A randomized controlled trial. *Obstetrics and Gynecology, 101*(2), 337–345.

Hall, E., Frey, B. N., & Soares, C. N. (2011). Non hormonal treatment strategies for vasomotor symptoms: A critical review. *Drugs, 71*(3), 287–304.

Heiss, G., Wallace, R., Anderson, G. L., Aragaki, A., Beresford, S. A., Brzyski, R., ... Stefanick, M. L. (2008). Health risks and benefits 3 years after stopping randomized treatment with estrogen and progestin. *The Journal of the American Medical Association, 299*(9), 1036–1045. doi:10.1001/jama.299.9.1036

Irvin, J. H., Domar, A. D., Clark, C., Zuttemzeister, P. C., & Friedman, R. (1996). The effects of relaxation response training on menopausal symptoms. *Journal of Psychosomatic Obstetrics and Gynaecology, 17*(4), 202–207.

Joffe, H., Partridge, A., Giobbie-Hurder, A., Li, X., Habin, K., Goss, P., ... Garber, J. (2010). Augmentation of venlafaxine and selective serotonin reuptake inhibitors with zolpidem improves sleep and quality of life in breast cancer patients with hot flashes: A randomized, double-blind, placebo-controlled trial. *Menopause, 17*(5), 908–916.

Kimmick, G. G., Lovato, J., McQuellon, R., Robinson, E., & Muss, H. B. (2006). Randomized, double–blind, placebo–controlled, crossover study of sertraline (zoloft) for the treatment of hot flashes in women with early stage breast cancer taking tamoxifen. *The Breast Journal, 12*(2), 114–122.

Lee, M. S., Kim, K. H., Choi, S. M., & Ernst, E. (2009). Acupuncture for treating hot flashes in breast cancer patients: A systematic review. *Breast Cancer Research and Treatment, 115*(3), 497–503.

Lee, M. S., Kim, J. I., Ha, J. Y., Boddy, K., & Ernst, E. (2009). Yoga for menopausal symptoms: A systematic review. *Menopause, 16*(3), 602–608.

Lee, M. S., Shin, B. C., & Ernst, E. (2009). Acupuncture for treating menopausal hot flushes: A systematic review. *Climacteric, 12*(1), 16–25.

Lengacher, C. A., Reich, R. R., Post-White, J., Moscoso, M., Shelton, M. M., Barta, M., ... Budhrani, P. (2012). Mindfulness-based stress reduction in post-treatment breast cancer patients: An examination of symptoms and symptom clusters. *Journal of Behavioral Medicine, 35*(1), 86–94.

Lewis, J. E., Nickell, L. A., Thompson, L. U., Szalai, J. P., Kiss, A., & Hilditch, J. R. (2006). A randomized controlled trial of the effect of dietary soy and flaxseed muffins on quality of life and hot flashes during menopause. *Menopause, 13*(4), 631–642.

Loprinzi, C. L., Kugler, J. W., Sloan, J. A., Mailliard, J. A., LaVasseur, B. I., Barton, D. L., ... Christensen, B. J. (2000). Venlafaxine in management of hot flashes in survivors of breast cancer: A randomised controlled trial. *The Lancet, 356*(9247), 2059–2063.

Loprinzi, C. L., Michalak, J. C., Quella, S. K., O'Fallon, J. R., Hatfield, A. K., Nelimark, R. A., ... Oesterling, J. E. (1994). Megestrol acetate for the prevention of hot flashes. *The New England Journal of Medicine, 331*(6), 347–352.

Loprinzi, C. L., Pisansky, T. M., Fonseca, R., Sloan, J. A., Zahasky, K. M., Quella, S. K., ... Perez, E. A. (1998). Pilot evaluation of venlafaxine hydrochloride for the therapy of hot flashes in cancer survivors. *Journal of Clinical Oncology, 16*(7), 2377–2381.

Loprinzi, C. L., Sloan, J. A., Perez, E. A., Quella, S. K., Stella, P. J., Mailliard, J. A., ... Rummans, T. A. (2002). Phase III evaluation of fluoxetine for treatment of hot flashes. *Journal of Clinical Oncology, 20*(6), 1578–1583.

Loprinzi, C. L., Sloan, J. A., Stearns, V., Slack, R., Iyengar, M., Diekmann, B., … Novotny, P. (2009). Newer antidepressants and gabapentin for hot flashes: An individual patient pooled analysis. *J Clin Oncol, 27*(17), 2831–2837.

Manson, J. E., Hsia, J., Johnson, K. C., Rossouw, J. E., Assaf, A. R., Lasser, N. L., … Cushman, M. (2003). Estrogen plus progestin and the risk of coronary heart disease. *The New England Journal of Medicine, 349*(6), 523–534.

Nelson, H. D., Vesco, K. K., Haney, E., Fu, R., Nedrow, A., Miller, J., … Humphrey, L. (2006). Nonhormonal therapies for menopausal hot flashes: Systematic review and meta-analysis. *The Journal of the American Medical Association, 295*(17), 2057–2071.

Pandya, K. J., Morrow, G. R., Roscoe, J. A., Zhao, H., Hickok, J. T., Pajon, E., … Flynn, P. J. (2005). Gabapentin for hot flashes in 420 women with breast cancer: A randomised double-blind placebo-controlled trial. *The Lancet, 366*(9488), 818–824.

Pandya, K. J., Raubertas, R. F., Flynn, P. J., Hynes, H. E., Rosenbluth, R. J., Kirshner, J. J., … Morrow, G. R. (2000). Oral clonidine in postmenopausal patients with breast cancer experiencing tamoxifen-induced hot flashes: A University of Rochester Cancer Center Community Clinical Oncology Program study. *Annals of Internal Medicine, 132*(10), 788–793.

Pockaj, B. A., Gallagher, J. G., Loprinzi, C. L., Stella, P. J., Barton, D. L., Sloan, J. A., … Fauq, A. H. (2006). Phase III double-blind, randomized, placebo-controlled crossover trial of black cohosh in the management of hot flashes: NCCTG Trial N01CC1. *Journal of Clinical Oncology, 24*(18), 2836–2841.

Quella, S. K., Loprinzi, C. L., Sloan, J. A., Vaught, N. L., DeKrey, W. L., Fischer, T., … Pisansky, T. (1998). Long-term use of megestrol acetate by cancer survivors for the treatment of hot flashes. *Cancer, 82*(9), 1784–1788.

Rahimi, R., & Abdollahi, M. (2012). An update on the ability of St. John's wort to affect the metabolism of other drugs. *Expert Opinion on Drug Metabolism and Toxicology, 8*(6), 691–708.

Reddy, S. Y., Warner, H., Guttuso, T., Jr., Messing, S., DiGrazio, W., Thornburg, L., & Guzick, D. S. (2006). Gabapentin, estrogen, and placebo for treating hot flushes: A randomized controlled trial. *Obstetrics and Gynecology, 108*(1), 41–48.

Rossouw, J. E., Anderson, G. L., Prentice, R. L., LaCroix, A. Z., Kooperberg, C., Stefanick, M. L., … Ockene, J. (2002). Risks and benefits of estrogen plus progestin in healthy postmenopausal women: Principal results from the Women's Health Initiative randomized controlled trial. *The Journal of the American Medical Association, 288*(3), 321–333.

Schober, C. E., & Ansani, N. T. (2003). Venlafaxine hydrochloride for the treatment of hot flashes. *The Annals of Pharmacotherapy, 37*(11), 1703–1707.

Shams, T., Setia, M. S., Hemmings, R., McCusker, J., Sewitch, M., & Ciampi, A. (2010). Efficacy of black cohosh-containing preparations on menopausal symptoms: A meta-analysis. *Alternative Therapy and Health Medicine, 16*(1), 36–44.

Simbalista, R. L., Sauerbronn, A. V., Aldrighi, J. M., & Arêas, J. A. (2010). Consumption of a flaxseed-rich food is not more effective than a placebo in alleviating the climacteric symptoms of postmenopausal women. *Journal of Nutrition, 140*(2), 293–297.

Smith, K. B., & Pukall, C. F. (2009). An evidence–based review of yoga as a complementary intervention for patients with cancer. *Psycho–Oncology, 18*(5), 465–475.

Stearns, V., Beebe, K. L., Iyengar, M., & Dube, E. (2003). Paroxetine controlled release in the treatment of menopausal hot flashes: A randomized controlled trial. *The Journal of the American Medical Association, 289*(21), 2827–2834.

Stearns, V., Isaacs, C., Rowland, J., Crawford, J., Ellis, M. J., Kramer, R., ... Hayes, D. F. (2000). A pilot trial assessing the efficacy of paroxetine hydrochloride (Paxil®) in controlling hot flashes in breast cancer survivors. *Annals of Oncology, 11*(1), 17–22.

Stearns, V., Slack, R., Greep, N., Henry-Tilman, R., Osborne, M., Bunnell, C., ... Isaacs, C. (2005). Paroxetine is an effective treatment for hot flashes: Results from a prospective randomized clinical trial. *Journal of Clinical Oncology, 23*(28), 6919–6930.

Suvanto-Luukkonen, E., Koivunen, R., Sundström, H., Bloigu, R., Karjalainen, E., Häivä-Mällinen, L., & Tapanainen, J. S. (2005). Citalopram and fluoxetine in the treatment of postmenopausal symptoms: A prospective, randomized, 9-month, placebo-controlled, double-blind study. *Menopause, 12*(1), 18–26.

Taku, K., Melby, M. K., Kronenberg, F., Kurzer, M. S., & Messina, M. (2012). Extracted or synthesized soybean isoflavones reduce menopausal hot flash frequency and severity: Systematic review and meta-analysis of randomized controlled trials. *Menopause, 19*(7), 776–790.

Tremblay, A., Sheeran, L., & Aranda, S. K. (2008). Psychoeducational interventions to alleviate hot flashes: A systematic review. *Menopause, 15*(1), 193–202.

Utian, W. H., Bachmann, G. A., Cahill, E. B., Gallagher, J. C., Grodstein, F., Heiman, J. R., ... Wysocki, S. (2010). Estrogen and progestogen use in postmenopausal women: 2010 position statement of The North American Menopause Society. *Menopause, 17*(2), 242–255.

van der Sluijs, C. P., Bensoussan, A., Chang, S., & Baber, R. (2009). A randomized placebo-controlled trial on the effectiveness of an herbal formula to alleviate menopausal vasomotor symptoms. *Menopause, 16*(2), 336–344.

Walker, E. M., Rodriguez, A. I., Kohn, B., Ball, R. M., Pegg, J., Pocock, J. R., ... Levine, R. A. (2010). Acupuncture versus venlafaxine for the management of vasomotor symptoms in patients with hormone receptor–positive breast cancer: A randomized controlled trial. *Journal of Clinical Oncology, 28*(4), 634–640.

Wassertheil-Smoller, S., Hendrix, S. L., Limacher, M., Heiss, G., Kooperberg, C., Baird, A., ... Mysiw, W. J. (2003). Effect of estrogen plus progestin on stroke in postmenopausal women: The Women's Health Initiative: A randomized trial. *The Journal of the American Medical Association, 289*(20), 2673–2684.

Weitzner, M. A., Moncello, J., Jacobsen, P. B., & Minton, S. (2002). A pilot trial of paroxetine for the treatment of hot flashes and associated symptoms in women with breast cancer. *Journal of Pain and Symptom Management, 23*(4), 337–345.

Williamson, J., White, A., Hart, A., & Ernst, E. (2002). Randomised controlled trial of reflexology for menopausal symptoms. *The British Journal of Obstetrics and Gynaecology, 109*(9), 1050–1055.

Witek-Janusek, L., Albuquerque, K., Chroniak, K. R., Chroniak, C., Durazo-Arvizu, R., & Mathews, H. L. (2008). Effect of mindfulness-based stress reduction on immune function, quality of life, and coping in women newly diagnosed with early stage breast cancer. *Brain, Behavior and Immunity*, *22*(6), 969–981.

Wu, J., Schneider, B., Ryker, K., & Tallman, E. (2013). Paced respiration for vasomotor and other menopausal symptoms: a randomized, controlled trial. *Journal of General Internal Medicine*, *28*(2), 193–200.

Ziaei, S., Kazemnejad, A., & Zareai, M. (2007). The effect of vitamin E on hot flashes in menopausal women. *Gynecology and Obstetrics Investigation*, *64*(4), 204–207.

CHAPTER 5

Cedars, M. I., & Evans, M. (2008). Menopause. In R. S. Gibbs, B. Y. Karlan, A. F. Haney, I. Nygaard (Eds.), *Danforth's obstetrics and gynecology* (10th ed., pp. 725–741). Philadelphia, PA: Lippincott Williams and Wilkins.

de Abajo, F. J., & Garcia-Rodriguez, L. A. (2008). Risk of upper gastrointestinal tract bleeding associated with selective serotonin reuptake inhibitors and venlafaxine therapy: Interaction with nonsteroidal anti-inflammatory drugs and effect of acid-suppressing agents. *Archives of General Psychiatry*, *65*(7), 795–803.

Fisher, W. I., Johnson, A. K., Elkins, G. R., Otte, J. L., Burns, D. S., Yu, M., & Carpenter, J. S. (2013). Risk factors, pathophysiology, and treatment of hot flashes in cancer. *CA: A Cancer Journal for Clinicians*, *63*(3), 167–192.

Richards, J. B., Papaioannou, A., Adachi, J. D., Joseph, L., Whitson, H. E., Prior, J. C., & Goltzman, D. (2007). Effect of selective serotonin reuptake inhibitors on the risk of fracture. *Archives of Internal Medicine*, *167*(2), 188–194.

Santoro, N. F. (2004). Treatment of menopause-associated vasomotor symptoms: Position statement of the North American menopause society. *Menopause*, *11*(1), 11–33.

Sicat, B. L., & Brokaw, D. K. (2004). Nonhormonal alternatives for the treatment of hot flashes. *Pharmacotherapy*, *24*(1), 79–93.

Stearns, V., Beebe, K. L., Iyengar, M., & Dube, E. (2003). Paroxetine-controlled release in the treatment of menopausal hot flashes: A randomized controlled trial. *The Journal of the American Medical Association*, *289*(21), 2827–2834.

CHAPTER 6

Elkins, G., Fisher, W., Johnson, A., Carpenter, J., & Keith, T. (2013). Clinical hypnosis in the treatment of postmenopausal hot flashes: A randomized controlled trial. *Menopause*, *20*(3), 291–298.

Elkins, G., Johnson A., Fisher, W., Slinwinski J. (2012). Improving sleep in post-menopausal women: Outcome from a randomized clinical trial. *Menopause*, *19*(12), 1371 (S-3).

Elkins, G., Marcus, J, Stearns, V., Perfect, M., Rajab, M. H., Ruud, C., ... Keith, T. (2008). Randomized trial of a hypnosis intervention for treatment of hot flashes among breast cancer survivors. *Journal of Clinical Oncology, 26* (31), 5022–5026.

Elkins, G., Sliwinski, J., Johnson, A., & Fisher, W. (2012). Guided self-hypnosis for the control of hot flashes: A pilot study. *Menopause, 19*(12), 1387 (P-32).

Elkins, G., Stearns, V., Marcus, J., & Rajab, H. (2007). Pilot evaluation of hypnosis for treatment of hot flashes in breast cancer survivors. *Psycho-Oncology, 16*(5), 487–492.

CHAPTER 7

Sloan, J. A., Loprinzi, C. L., Novotny, P. J., Barton, D. L., Lavasseur, B. I., & Windschitl, H. (2001). Methodologic lessons learned from hot flash studies. *Journal of Clinical Oncology, 19*(23), 4280–4290.

CHAPTER 8

Elkins, G., Marcus, J., Stearns, V., & Hasan Rajab, M. (2007). Pilot evaluation of hypnosis for the treatment of hot flashes in breast cancer survivors. *Psycho-Oncology, 6*(5), 487–492.

Mohyi, D., Tabassi, K., & Simon, J. (1997). Differential diagnosis of hot flashes. *Maturitas, 27*, 203–214.

Stearns, V., Ullmer, L., Lopez, J. F., Smith, Y., Isaacs, C., & Hayes, D. F. (2002). Hot flushes. *The Lancet, 360*(9348), 1851–1861.

CHAPTER 9

Buysse, D. J., Yu, L., Moul, D. E., Germain, A., Stover, A., Dodds, N. E., ... Pilkonis, P. A. (2010). Development and validation of patient-reported outcome measures for sleep disturbance and sleep-related impairments. *Sleep, 33*(6), 781–792.

Davidson, J. R. (2013). Sink into sleep. New York, NY: Demos Medical.

Dennerstein, L., Lehert, P., Guthrie, J. R., & Burger, H. G. (2007). Modeling women's health during the menopausal transition: A longitudinal analysis. *Menopause, 14*(1), 53–62.

Kravitz, H. M., Ganz, P. A., Bromberger, J., Powell, L. H., Sutton-Tyrrel, K., & Meyer, P. M. (2003). Sleep difficulty in women at midlife: A community survey of sleep and the menopausal transition. *Menopause, 10*(1), 19–28.

NIH State-of-the-Science Panel. (2005). National Institutes of Health State-of-the Science conference statement: Management of menopause-related symptoms. *Annals of Internal Medicine, 142*(12), 1003–1013.

CHAPTER 10

Carpenter, J. S. (2001). The hot flash related daily interference scale: A tool for assessing the impact of hot flashes on quality of life following breast cancer. *Journal of Pain and Symptom Management, 22*(6), 979–989.

daCosta DiBonaventura, M., Wagner, J. S., Alvir, J., & Whiteley, J. (2012). Depression, quality of life, work productivity, resource use, and costs among women experiencing menopause and hot flashes: A cross-sectional study. *The Primary Care Companion for CNS Disorders, 14*(6), doi:10.4088/PCC.12m01410

Freeman, E. W., Sammel, M. D., Lin, H., Gracia, C. R., Kapoor, S., & Ferdousi, T. (2005). The role of anxiety and hormonal changes in menopausal hot flashes. *Menopause, 12*(3), 258–266.

Mood. (n.d.). *In Merriam-Webster Dictionary online.* Retrieved from www.merriam-webster.com/dictionary/mood

Thurston, R. C., Blumenthal, J. A., Babyak, M. A., & Sherwood, A. (2005). Emotional antecedents of hot flashes during daily life. *Psychosomatic Medicine, 67,* 137–146.

CHAPTER 11

Crasilneck, H., & Hall, J. (1985). *Clinical hypnosis: Principles and applications.* Boston, MA: Allyn and Bacon.

Elkins, G. (2013). *Hypnotic relaxation therapy: Principles and applications.* New York, NY: Springer Publishing.

Hartland, J. (1979). *Medical and dental hypnosis and its clinical applications.* Baltimore, MD: Williams & Wilkins Company.

Kroger, W. (1977). *Clinical and experimental hypnosis in medicine, dentistry, and psychology.* Philadelphia, PA: J.B. Lippincott Company.

CHAPTER 18

American Society of Clinical Hypnosis. (1990). Hypnosis with sexual dysfunction and relationship problems. In D. C. Hammond (Ed.), *Handbook of hypnotic suggestions and metaphors* (1st ed., pp. 349–370). New York, NY: WW Norton & Company.

Bancroft, J. (2005). The endocrinology of sexual arousal. *Journal of Endocrinology, 186*(3), 411–427.

Basson, R. (2006). The complexities of women's sexuality and the menopause transition. *Menopause, 13*(6), 853–855.

Biglia, N., Moggio, G., Peano, E., Sgandurra, P., Ponzone, R., Nappi, R. E., & Sismondi, P. (2010). Effects of surgical and adjuvant therapies for breast cancer on sexuality, cognitive functions, and body weight. *The Journal of Sexual Medicine, 7*(5), 1891–1900.

Brotto, L. A., Erskine, Y., Carey, M., Ehlen, T., Finlayson, S., Heywood, M., … Miller, D. (2012). A brief mindfulness-based cognitive behavioral intervention improves sexual functioning versus wait-list control in women treated for gynecologic cancer. *Gynecologic Oncology, 125*(2), 320–325.

Burwell, S. R., Case, L. D., Kaelin, C., & Avis, N. E. (2006). Sexual problems in younger women after breast cancer surgery. *Journal of Clinical Oncology, 24*(18), 2815–2821.

Cyranowski, J. M., Aarestad, S. L., & Andersen, B. L. (1999). The role of sexual self-schema in a diathesis-stress model of sexual dysfunction. *Applied and Preventative Psychology, 8*(3), 217–228.

Cyranowski, J. M., & Andersen, B. L. (1998). Schemas, sexuality, and romantic attachment. *Journal of Personality and Social Psychology, 74*(5), 1364–1379.

Cyranowski, J. M., & Andersen, B. L. (2000). Evidence of self-schematic cognitive processing in women with differing sexual self-views. *Journal of Social and Clinical Psychology, 19*(4), 519–543.

Davis, M. W. (2003). *The sex-starved marriage: Boosting your marriage libido.* New York, NY: Simon & Schuster.

de Luque, P. J., Jiménez, A. M., Alvarado, M. A., Jiménez, P. B., & Inchausti, F. S. (2009). Sexuality during menopause. *Revista de Enfermería, 32*(11), 52–57.

Dennerstein, L. (2008). Sexuality, midlife, and menopause. *Menopause, 15*(2), 221–222.

Elkins, G. R., Fisher, W. I., Johnson, A. K., Carpenter, J. S., & Keith, T. Z. (2013). Clinical hypnosis in the treatment of postmenopausal hot flashes: A randomized controlled trial. *Menopause, 20*(3), 291–298.

Emilee, G., Ussher, J. M., & Perz, J. (2010). Sexuality after breast cancer: A review. *Maturitas, 66*(4), 397–407.

Firestone, R., Firestone, L., & Catlett, J. (2006). *Sex and love in intimate relationships.* Washington, DC: American Psychological Association.

Fobair, P., & Spiegel, D. (2009). Concerns about sexuality after breast cancer. *The Cancer Journal, 15*(1), 19–26.

Foley, S., Kope, S. A., & Sugrue, D. P. (2002). *Sex matters for women: A complete guide to taking care of your sexual self.* New York, NY: Guilford Press.

Frierson, G. M., Thiel, D. L., & Andersen, B. L. (2006). Body change stress for women with breast cancer: The Breast-Impact of Treatment Scale. *Annals of Behavioral Medicine, 32*(1), 77–81.

Frohlich, J., Ogawa, S., Morgan, M., Burton, L., & Pfaff, D. (1999). Hormones, genes, and the structure of sexual arousal. *Behavioral Brain Research, 105*(1), 5–27.

Ganz, P. A., Desmond, K. A., Belin, T. R., Meyerowitz, B. E., & Rowland, J. H. (1999). Predictors of sexual health in women after a breast cancer diagnosis. *Journal of Clinical Oncology, 17*(8), 2371–2380.

Ganz, P. A., Greendale, G. A., Petersen, L., Kahn, B., & Bower, J. E. (2003). Breast cancer in younger women: Reproductive and late health effects of treatment. *Journal of Clinical Oncology, 21*(22), 4184–4193.

Ganz, P. A., Rowland, J. H., Desmond, K., Meyerowitz, B. E., & Wyatt, G. E.(1998). Life after breast cancer: Understanding women's health-related quality of life and sexual functioning. *Journal of Clinical Oncology, 16*(2), 501–514.

Genazzani, A. R., Gambacciani, M., & Simoncini, T. (2007). Menopause and aging, quality of life and sexuality. *Climacteric, 10*(2), 88–96.

Goldstein, S. W., & Arleque, L. (2007). *When sex isn't good: Stories & solutions of women with sexual dysfunction.* Bloomington, IN: iUniverse.

Gottman, J. (1994). *Why marriages succeed or fail: And how you can make yours last.* New York, NY: Simon & Schuster.

Gottman, J., & Silver, N. (1999). *The seven principles for making marriage work.* Hoboken, NJ: John Wiley & Sons.

Graziottin, A. (2007). Effect of premature menopause on sexuality. *Women's Health (London England), 3*(4), 455–474.

Graziottin, A. (2010). Menopause and sexuality: Key issues in premature menopause and beyond. *Annals of the New York Academy of Sciences, 1205,* 254–261.

Grio, R., Cellura, A., Porpiglia, M., Geranio, R., & Piacentino, R. (1999). Sexuality in menopause: Importance of adequate replacement therapy. *Minerva Ginecologica, 51*(3), 59–62.

Hernández, L. E., Hernández, M. V., Diéguez, M. J. M., & Rodríguez, A. R. (2013). Changes in sexuality during menopause. *Atención Primaria, 45*(6), 329–330.

Hull, E. M., Lorrain, D. S., Du, J., Matuszewich, L., Lumley, L. A., Putnam, S. K., & Moses, J. (1999). Hormone–neurotransmitter interactions in the control of sexual behavior. *Behavioral Brain Research, 105*(1), 105–116.

Jun, E. Y., Kim, S., Chang, S. B., Oh, K., Kang, H. S., & Kang, S. S. (2011). The effect of a sexual life reframing program on marital intimacy, body image, and sexual function among breast cancer survivors. *Cancer Nursing, 34*(2), 142–149.

Kalaitzi, C., Papadopoulos, V. P., Michas, K., Vlasis, K., Skandalakis, P., & Filippou, D. (2007). Combined brief psychosexual intervention after mastectomy: Effects on sexuality, body image, and psychological well–being. *Journal of Surgical Oncology, 96*(3), 235–240.

Karaöz, B., Aksu, H., & Küçük, M. (2010). A qualitative study of the information needs of premenopausal women with breast cancer in terms of contraception, sexuality, early menopause, and fertility. *International Journal of Gynaecology and Obstetrics, 109*(2), 118–120.

Lin, H., & Mogul, M. (2007). Hormones and sexuality during transition to menopause. *Obstetrics and Gynecology, 109*(4), 831–840.

Lo, S. S., & Kok, W. M. (2013). Sexuality of Chinese women around menopause. *Maturitas, 74*(2), 190–195.

Mann, E., Smith, M. J., Hellier, J., Balabanovic, J. A., Hamed, H., Grunfeld, E. A., & Hunter, M. S. (2012). Cognitive behavioural treatment for women who have menopausal symptoms after breast cancer treatment (MENOS 1): A randomised controlled trial. *The Lancet Oncology, 13*(3), 309–318.

McCarthy, B., & McCarthy, E. (2003). *Rekindling desire: A step-by-step program to help low-sex and no-sex marriages.* New York, NY: Routledge.

McCoy, N. L. (2002). Longitudinal study of menopause and sexuality. *Acta Obstetricia et Gynecologica Scandinavica, 81*(7), 617–622.

Nappi, R. E. (2007). New attitudes to sexuality in the menopause: clinical evaluation and diagnosis. *Climacteric, 10*(2), 105–108.

Nappi, R. E., & Lachowsky, M. (2009). Menopause and sexuality: Prevalence of symptoms and impact on quality of life. *Maturitas, 63*(2), 138–141.

Nappi, R. E., & Nijland, E. A. (2008). Women's perception of sexuality around the menopause: Outcomes of a European telephone survey. *European Journal of Obstetrics and Gynecology Reproductive Biology, 137*(1), 10–16.

NIH State-of-the-Science Panel. (2005). National Institutes of Health State-of-the-Science Conference statement: management of menopause-related symptoms. *Annals of Internal Medicine, 142*, 1003–1013.

Pitkin, J. (2009). Sexuality and the menopause. *Best Practice and Research Clinical Obstetrics and Gynaecology, 23*(1), 33–52.

Rogers, M., & Kristjanson, L. J. (2002). The impact on sexual functioning of chemotherapy-induced menopause in women with breast cancer. *Cancer Nursing, 25*(1), 57–65.

Rowland, J. H., Meyerowitz, B. E., Crespi, C. M., Leedham, B., Desmond, K., Belin, T. R., & Ganz, P. A. (2009). Addressing intimacy and partner communication after breast cancer: A randomized controlled group intervention. *Breast Cancer Research and Treatment, 118*(1), 99–111.

Safarinejad, M. R. (2011). Reversal of SSRI-induced female sexual dysfunction by adjunctive bupropion in menstruating women: A double-blind, placebo-controlled and randomized study. *Journal of Psychopharmacology, 25*(3), 370–378.

Segraves, T., Croft, H., Kavoussi, R., Ascher, J. A., Batey, S. R., Foster, V. J., ... Metz, A. R. (2001). Bupropion sustained release (SR) for the treatment of hypoactive sexual desire disorder (HSDD) in nondepressed women. *Journal of Sex and Marital Therapy, 27*(3), 303–316.

Shifren, J. L., & Avis, N. E. (2007). Surgical menopause: effects on psychological well-being and sexuality. *Menopause, 14*(3 pt 2), 586–591.

van Anders, S. M. (2012). Testosterone and sexual desire in healthy women and men. *Archives of Sexual Behavior, 41*(6), 1471–1484.

von Sydow, K. (2000). Sexuality of older women. The effect of menopause, other physical and social and partner related factors. *German Journal for Quality in Health Care, 94*(3), 223–229.

Wilmoth, M. C., Coleman, E. A., Smith, S. C., & Davis, C. (2004). Fatigue, weight gain, and altered sexuality in patients with breast cancer: Exploration of a symptom cluster. In *Oncology Nursing Forum, 51* (6), 1069–1075.

Wylie, K. R. (2006). Sexuality and the menopause. *Journal of the British Menopause Society, 12*(4), 149–152.

Young-McCaughan, S. (1996). Sexual functioning in women with breast cancer after treatment with adjuvant therapy. *Cancer Nursing, 19*(4), 308–319.

Index

achieving hypnotic relaxation, 120
acupuncture, 55
aerobic exercise, 57
alcohol, as hot flash trigger, 89
alternative medicine therapies.
        See also herbal and
        nonprescription remedies
    acupuncture, 55
    biofeedback and relaxation
        training, 51–52
    exercise, 56–57
    magnet therapy, 57
    mindfulness-based stress
        reduction, 57–58
    paced respiration, 58
    psychoeducation and cognitive-
        behavioral programs, 59
    reflexology, 59
    yoga, 60–61
American Society of Clinical
        Hypnosis (ASCH), 214
antidepressants, 46
    citalopram, 47
    fluoxetine, 48
    paroxetine, 47–48
    side effects of, 46
    venlafaxine, 47
anxiety, 4, 20, 29, 88, 102
    and benefits of hormone
        therapy, 38
ASCH. *See* American Society of
        Clinical Hypnosis
audio recordings
    beginning with, 122–124

*Hypnotic Relaxation for Hot Flashes:
        Awareness and Control*, 163,
        171–174, 188–189
*Hypnotic Relaxation Therapy for Hot
        Flashes-Lake Imagery*, 119–120,
        141, 158, 188–189
*Hypnotic Relaxation Therapy for
        Hot Flashes-Mountain Imagery*,
        119–120, 141, 158, 188–189
*Individualizing Hypnotic Relaxation
        for Hot Flashes*, 137–141, 158,
        188–189
Learning Self-Hypnosis, 141,
        155–158
    regular practice with, 209–210
    ten steps to successful practice,
        122, 139, 156, 172, 188
    what to expect on, 120–121,
        137–139, 154–157, 171–172
autonomic nervous system (ANS), 112

Bellergal, 49
biofeedback therapy, 55–56
Biolog, 16
Biolog recorders, 69
black cohosh, 51
blood clots, as risk of
        hormone therapy, 39
Braid, James, 66
"brain fog," 30
breast cancer, 23–24
    "brain fog" and concentration, 30
    diagnosis and stage, 27–29

breast cancer (*cont.*)
  emotional, cognitive, and
      relational impact of, 29–31
  hypnotic relaxation among
      survivors, 26–27
  interpersonal relationships, impact
      on, 30–31
  risk for depression, 29–30
  as risk of hormone therapy, 39
  support and coping with
      adjustment issues,
          recognized, 31
      counseling, 32
      self-care and emotional
          support, 32
      sharing feelings to relieve
          stress, 31–32
  treatment, 24–26
      chemotherapy, 24
      radiation therapy, 25
      surgery, 24
      tamoxifen and raloxifene, 25
Brisdelle (paroxetine), 47–48

calmness, 115
Canadian Society of Hypnosis
    (CSH), 215
cancer treatment and hot flashes,
    24–26
cardiovascular disease, as risk of
    hormone therapy, 39
Charcot, Jean Marie, 66
chemotherapy, breast cancer
    treatment, 24
Cimicifuga racemosa, 51
citalopram. *See* Lexapro
clonidine, 49
cognitive-behavioral programs, 59
colorectal cancer, and benefits of
    hormone therapy, 38
conscious alertness, 116
conscious level of awareness, 68
"control condition," 26
coolness, 116

Coumadin, 48
counseling
  for emotional concerns, 32
  hypnotic relaxation therapy
      versus, 69
counting hot flashes, strategies for,
    84–85
CSH. *See* Canadian Society of
    Hypnosis

deep venous thrombosis
    (DVT), 39
depression. *See also* breast cancer
  clinical, 29–30
  and effect on hypnotic relaxation
      therapy, 213
  and hot flashes, 102
dong quai, 51
drugs, as hot flash triggers, 89

Effexor (venlafaxine), 55, 47
Emily
  background, 81
  how Emily did on the program,
      201–203
  Hot Flash Daily Diaries, 82–83,
      133, 151, 167, 183
  Hot Flash Related Daily
      Interference Scale (HFRDIS),
      107, 207
  Hot Flash Score reduction
      percentages, 132, 150, 166,
      182, 201
  Hot Flash Relaxation Practice
      Checklist, 134–135, 152–153,
      168–169, 184–185
  identifying triggers, 89–90, 91, 92
  individualized images,
      136–137, 138
  rating interference of hot flashes,
      104–106
  Sleep Rating Form, 98, 99
emotional relaxation, 47

emotional support, 32
endometrial cancer, as risk of
    hormone therapy, 40
environment, as hot flash trigger,
    89–90
estrogen plus progestin therapy
    (EPT), 35
estrogen therapy (ET), 35
Evista. *See* raloxifene
exercise, 56–57

flax seed, 48
fluoxetine. *See* Prozac
Food and Drug Administration
    (FDA), 46
foods, as hot flash triggers, 89
foot reflexology, 59
Franklin, Benjamin, 65
Freud, Sigmund, 66

gabapentin, 49–50
ginseng, 52

Hatha yoga, 60
herbal and nonprescription
    remedies, 50–51. *See also*
    alternative medicine therapies
  black cohosh, 51
  dong quai, 51
  evening primrose, 51–52
  flax seed, 52
  ginseng, 52
  red clover, 52–53
  soy isoflavones, 53
  St. John's wort, 53–54
  vitamin E, 54
HFRDIS. *See* Hot Flash Related Daily
    Interference Scale
hip fractures, and benefits of
    hormone therapy, 38
hormone replacement therapy.
    See hormone therapy

hormone therapy (HT), 3, 33–34,
    41–42
  benefits of menopausal, 37, 40–41
  forms of menopausal, 34–35
  questions for your doctor, 42
  reconsidered, 35–37
  risks of menopausal
    blood clots, 39
    breast cancer, 39
    cardiovascular disease, 39
    endometrial cancer, 40
    stroke, 40
  types of, 34–35
  weighing risks and benefits,
    40–41
  who should not use, 41–42
Hot Flash Daily Diary, 76–77, 86,
    126, 143, 160, 176, 191. *See also*
    Emily; *Relief from Hot Flashes*
    program
  baseline, 76, 85–86
  counting hot flashes, 84–85
  getting started, 75–76, 77–81, 83
  reviewing, 130–131, 147–149,
    164–165, 180–181, 196–197
hot flashes, 116. *See also, Relief from
    Hot Flashes* program
  alternative therapies for,
    54–59
  among women during
    menopausal transition, 4
  antidepressants for, 20, 46–48
  benefits of hormone therapy, 37
  cancer treatment and, 22–26
  changes in body during,
    15–18
  discuss issues with doctor, 13
  effect on
    mood, 101–102
    quality of life, 99–100
    relationships, 102–103
  frequency by objective
    measurement, 17
  herbal and nonprescription drugs
    for, 50–54

hot flashes (*cont.*)
   hypnotic relaxation therapy for, 3,
      5, 8, 26–27
   medication for, 13
   in men, 20–21
   other prescription drugs for, 48–50
   physiology of, 18–19
   psychology of, 19–20
   research on hypnotic relaxation
      therapy for, 68–70
   severity, 18, 78, 80
      definitions, 79
   and sleep, 95–96
   symptoms associated with, 4
Hot Flash Related Daily Interference
   Scale (HFRDIS), 108, 200.
   See also Emily
   described, 104
   using, 106, 199
hot flash score, 132, 163–166,
   181–182, 201. *See also* Emily
   calculating, 80–81, 83, 131 147–149,
     164–165, 180–181, 197
Hot Flash Triggers log, 93, 127, 144,
   161, 177, 192. *See also* Emily
   using, 125, 142, 159, 190
HT. *See* hormone therapy
Hypericum perforatum, 53
hypnosis. *See also*, self-hypnosis
   definition of hypnotic state, 64
   history of, 65–67
hypnotic abilities, 117–118
   achieving, 120–121, 171–172
   practice, 201–203, 213, 210
hypnotic relaxation for hot flashes,
   ten steps to successful practice
   of, 122, 139, 156, 172, 188
Hypnotic Relaxation Practice
   Checklist , 128, 145, 162, 178,
   193. *See also* Emily
   using, 125, 134, 142, 149, 152, 159,
   168, 175, 184, 190
hypnotic relaxation therapy, 3, 5, 125,
   56, 59, 167, 182. *See also*, *Relief
   from Hot Flashes* program

among breast cancer survivors,
   26–27
changes in sleep quality with, 10
and confidence, growth of, 117
definition, 64
and feeling less stress, 10–11
foundations, 67–68
goal, 64
history, 65
hypnotic abilities, 117–118
hypnotic state, 114–115
process of, 111–112
program, 150, 166
research on, 67–70
versus structured attention, 69
hypothalamus, 18

individualization, 136
individualized imagery, 11
individualized mental imagery,
   211–212
International Society of Hypnosis
   (ISH), 215
ISH. *See* International Society of
   Hypnosis
Iyengar yoga, 60

leisure activities, hot flashes
   effect on, 103
Lexapro (citalopram), 47
life ratings, mood, relationships, and
   quality of, 199
Linum usitatissimum, 52
locally applied estrogen, 35
lumpectomy, 24

magnet therapy, 57
major depression, 29
massage, 59
mastectomy, 24
MBSR. *See* mindfulness-based stress
   reduction

medication for hot flashes, 13
megestrol acetate, 50
men, hot flashes in, 20–21
menopausal transition, 96
  hot flashes among women
    during, 4
menopause, 95
  defined, 12
  and family and coworkers, 12
  symptoms of, 11–12
mental imagery, 11, 115, 121, 138, 172
  identification of individualized,
    211–212
Mesmer, Franz Anton, 65–66
mind–body therapy, 5, 64
mindfulness-based stress reduction
    (MBSR), 57–58
mood, hot flashes effect on,
    101–102, 106

nadis, 60
National Center for Complementary
    and Alternative Medicine
    (NCCAM), 8, 67
National Institutes of Health (NIH),
    8, 67
neutral zone, 18, 19
niacin, 89
"night sweats," 4
Nolvadex. See tamoxifen
nonhormonal therapies for hot
    flashes
  alternative medicine therapies.
  antidepressants, 46
  categories, 45–46
  herbals and nonprescription
    remedies, 50–51
  other prescription drugs, 48
nonprescription remedies, 50–51

Oenothera biennis, 51
On the Influence of the Planets on the
    Human Body (Mesmer), 65

paced respiration, 58
parasympathetic nervous system,
    113
paroxetine. See Paxil/Brisdelle
Paxil/Brisdelle (paroxetine),
    47–48
perimenopause, 11
"persistence pays off," 213
personal health care provider, 13
physiology of hot flashes, 18–19
postmenopause, 12
Premarin, 34
prescription drugs, as hot flash
    therapies, 48
  Bellergal, 49
  clonidine, 49
  gabapentin, 49–50
  megestrol acetate, 50
  Prozac (fluoxetine), 48
  psychoeducation, 59
  psychological stress, 88
  sleep loss associated with, 97
psychology of hot flashes, 19–20
pulmonary emboli (PE), 39

quality of life (QOL), 199, 203
  hot flashes effect on, 103–104, 106

radiation therapy, breast cancer
    treatment, 25
raloxifene (Evista), 25
red clover, 52–53
reflexology, 59
relationships
  breast cancer impact on, 30–31
  hot flashes effect on, 102, 106
relaxation, 10–11, 66
  training, 55–56
relaxation response, 113
Relief from Hot Flashes program.
    See also audio recordings;
    Emily; hypnotic relaxation
    therapy

Relief from Hot Flashes program.
(*cont.*)
about hot flashes, 3–5, 15–21
additional help, adjusting your
practice, 187
after completion of, 208
assessing your progress, 195–199
assessing your sleep, 95–98, 198
for breast cancer survivors,
26–27, 32
calculating your hot flash score,
80–81,
calculating reductions of hot flash
score, 148–149, 164–165,
180–181, 196–197
evidence for, 7–10
identifying hot flash triggers,
87–91
identifying the impacts of hot
flashes in your daily life,
101–104
improving daily practice, 170
individualizing your practice,
136–137, 211
maintaining your Hot Flash Daily
Diary, 124–125, 158, 174,
190, 211
making time and space to practice,
189, 210
not trying too hard, 212–213
overview of, 6–7
persistence, 213
practicing self-hypnosis,
154, 189, 212
the process of hypnotic relaxation,
111–118
recording your hot flashes, 83–85
reviewing and calculating your
hot flash scores, 130–131,
147–148, 163–165, 180–181
reviewing your hypnotic
relaxation practice checklist
and triggers, 134, 142, 168,
175, 184, 190, 210–211
weekly goals, 119, 186, 190
research on hypnotic relaxation
therapy, 68–70

safe place imagery, 115
SCEH. *See* Society for Clinical and
Experimental Hypnosis
selective estrogen-receptor
modulators (SERMs), 25
selective norepinephrine reuptake
inhibitors (SNRI), 47
selective serotonin reuptake
inhibitors (SSRI), 47–48
self-care, 32
self-hypnosis, 154. *See also* audio
recordings
effective use of, 212
skin temperature, during
hot flash, 16
sleep, 198, 202
assessing, 95–100
awareness of, 96
difficulties, 37
hot flashes and, 95–96
importance, 96–97
problems, 95
quality, 8–10
changes with hypnotic
relaxation, 10
Sleep Rating Form, 97–198, 206
using, 97–98, 198
social activities, hot flashes effect on,
103
Society for Clinical and Experimental
Hypnosis (SCEH), 214
Society for Psychological Hypnosis,
215
soy isoflavones, 53
SNRI. *See* selective norepinephrine
reuptake inhibitors
SSRI. *See* selective serotonin
reuptake inhibitors
St. John's wort, 53–54

stress, 20, 88, 101–102
  and emotional factors, 213
  stroke, as risk of hormone
    therapy, 40
surgery, breast cancer treatment, 24
sympathetic nervous system, 112

tamoxifen (Nolvadex), 25
TCM. *See* Traditional Chinese
    Medicine
ten steps to successful practice of
    hypnotic relaxation for hot
    flashes, 122, 139, 156,
    172, 188
Traditional Chinese Medicine
    (TCM), 51, 52
Trifolium pratense, 52
triggers
  changing/avoiding, 90–91
  identifying
    drugs/alcohol, 89
    emotional situations, 88

environment/activities, 89–90
  foods, 89
  stress/anxiety, 88
review, 210–211

unconscious levels of awareness, 68

vaginal dryness, benefits of hormone
    therapy, 38
venlafaxine. *See* Effexor
vitamin E, 54

Women's Health Initiative (WHI)
    study, 36–37

yoga, 60–61
  benefits, 60
  styles, 60

About the Author

Gary R. Elkins, PhD, ABPP, ABPH, is the Director of the Mind–Body Medicine Research Laboratory at Baylor University. He is a Professor of Psychology and Neuroscience at Baylor University where he is the Director of the Doctoral Program in Clinical Psychology. Dr. Elkins is also a Clinical Professor in the Texas A&M University Health Science Center. He maintains a private practice in clinical psychology with a specialization in clinical health psychology, behavioral medicine, and hypnotherapy. Dr. Elkins has board certification from the American Board of Professional Psychology (ABPP) and from the American Board of Psychological Hypnosis (ABPH). He is a Past-President of the American Society of Clinical Hypnosis and of the American Board of Psychological Hypnosis. He is the 2014 President of Division 30 (the Society of Psychological Hypnosis) of the American Psychological Association. With over 35 years of experience, he conducts an ongoing program of research into the use of hypnotic relaxation therapy and mind–body interventions for hot flashes, menopausal symptoms, and improving sleep. Dr. Elkins is the author of the groundbreaking publication *Hypnotic Relaxation Therapy: Principles and Applications* that provides a resource for training health care providers.

www.GaryElkins.org